The Health Improvement Profile (HIP)

Full the full range of M&K Publishing books please visit our website:
www.mkupdate.co.uk

The Health Improvement Profile (HIP)

■ ■ ■

A manual to promote physical wellbeing in people with severe mental illness

Sheila Hardy · Jacquie White · Richard Gray

The Health Improvement Profile (HIP)

A manual to promote physical wellbeing in people with severe mental illness

Sheila Hardy
Jacquie White
Richard Gray

ISBN: 9781905539918

First published 2015

British Library Catalogue in Publication Data
A catalogue record for this book is available from the British Library

Notice

Clinical practice and medical knowledge constantly evolve. Standard safety precautions must be followed, but, as knowledge is broadened by research, changes in practice, treatment and drug therapy may become necessary or appropriate. Readers must check the most current product information provided by the manufacturer of each drug to be administered and verify the dosages and correct administration, as well as contraindications. It is the responsibility of the practitioner, utilising the experience and knowledge of the patient, to determine dosages and the best treatment for each individual patient. Any brands mentioned in this book are as examples only and are not endorsed by the Publisher. Neither the publisher nor the authors assume any liability for any injury and/or damage to persons or property arising from this publication.

Disclaimer

M&K Publishing cannot accept responsibility for the contents of any linked website or online resource. The existence of a link does not imply any endorsement or recommendation of the organisation or the information or views which may be expressed in any linked website or online resource. We cannot guarantee that these links will operate consistently and we have no control over the availability of linked pages.

The Publisher

To contact M&K Publishing write to:
M&K Update Ltd · The Old Bakery · St. John's Street · Keswick · Cumbria CA12 5AS
Tel: 01768 773030 · Fax: 01768 781099
publishing@mkupdate.co.uk
www.mkupdate.co.uk

Designed and typeset by Mary Blood
Printed in Scotland by Bell & Bain

■ ■ ■ Contents

■ ■ ■ About the authors

Dr Sheila Hardy PhD MSc BSc NISP RMN RGN

Sheila is Senior Research Fellow at Northamptonshire Healthcare NHS Foundation Trust, Postgraduate Nurse Educator for the Charlie Waller Memorial Trust, Honorary Senior Lecturer at UCL and Visiting Fellow at the University of Northampton. She has twenty years of experience in primary care, where her clinical work included caring for patients with physical and mental health problems. Sheila is keen to improve the care of people with mental health issues and has carried out research and developed training in this area. Sheila sits on a number of national expert reference and steering groups.

Jacquie White RMN BSc (Hons) PGCert

Jacquie, a Registered Mental Health Nurse since 1986, studied the role of the mental health nurse in medication management on the acute unit for her first degree at the University of Hull in the 1990s. Developing practice that has an impact on the health of people with serious mental illness remains the focus of her teaching, research and scholarship. Jacquie has worked in the Faculty of Health and Social Care at the University of Hull since 2002, was promoted to Senior Lecturer in 2011 and is also Deputy Head of the Department of Psychological Health and Wellbeing.

Professor Richard J Gray BSc (Hons) MSc DLSHTM PhD RN FEANS

Richard trained at King's College London as a Mental Health Nurse and at the London School of Hygiene and Tropical Medicine in Public Health. He was awarded his PhD in 2001 from King's College London and in the same year was awarded a Medical Research Council Post Doctoral Fellowship. He was Professor of Research and Associate Dean at the University of East Anglia from 2008 to 2012. He currently leads a multidisciplinary Health Services Research group in Doha, Qatar, that does research on behaviour change, multi-morbidity and workforce. He is also Associate Editor of the *Journal of Psychiatric and Mental Health Nursing*. He has published more peer review papers than Professor Brian Cox but has never been invited to be a guest panellist on Radio 4's The Infinite Monkey Cage.

∎ ∎ ∎ Introduction

This book is intended as a practical guide to support healthcare practitioners in undertaking physical health checks for people with severe mental illness.

In people with severe mental illness (SMI), life expectancy is reduced by 12 to 19 years. The National Institute for Health and Care Excellence (NICE) in England therefore recommend that this group should receive a physical health check at least once a year. The major cause of death is cardiovascular disease (CVD) caused by a combination of unhealthy diet, lack of exercise and weight gain. Some of the antipsychotic medications used to treat patients with SMI have been implicated in raising this risk.

However, many mental health practitioners do not feel confident in assessing the physical health needs of people with SMI, as there is a lack of existing training in this subject. Even when training is offered, it is difficult for staff to access it because of their clinical workload commitments. The Health Improvement Profile (HIP) has therefore been created to assist healthcare practitioners in taking on this role effectively.

The HIP is an evidence-derived physical health check tool specifically designed to address all the physical health problems that are more common in people with SMI. It supports healthcare practitioners in identifying these physical health problems and guides them towards evidence-based interventions to address the problems.

What is severe mental illness?

Severe mental illness (SMI) is also known in the literature as severe and persistent mental illness or serious mental illness. It includes schizophrenia, bipolar disorder and other psychoses. In this chapter we talk about two main conditions (schizophrenia and bipolar disorder). Other psychoses include schizotypal personality, persistent delusional disorder, acute/transient psychotic disorders, induced delusional disorders, schizoaffective disorders, manic episodes, severe depression with psychosis and non-organic psychosis. These conditions are not explained individually in this book, as they all share symptoms with schizophrenia or bipolar disorder. Mental illnesses, such as depression and eating disorders, are not discussed either because the care of people with SMI is considered separately in United Kingdom (UK) guidance (NICE 2006, 2013, BMA and NHS Employers 2013).

■ ■ ■ Schizophrenia

Schizophrenia is a psychotic disorder characterised by positive, negative and cognitive symptoms (see Table 1.1). Positive symptoms include hallucinations (hearing voices or seeing visions), delusions (beliefs held strongly by the person but not shared by people around them) and thought disorder (for example, conversation jumping from one thought to another completely unrelated thought). Social isolation and withdrawal are examples of negative symptoms.

Cognitive symptoms are very common and include problems with concentration and planning tasks. Schizophrenia is a long-term condition and life expectancy is reduced by around 20 years compared to the general population (Wahlbeck et al. 2011). About two-thirds of excess mortality is due to natural causes, including cardiovascular disease, cancer, respiratory, and lung diseases (Colton & Manderscheid 2006). The symptoms of schizophrenia often result in major social or occupational disturbance. For example, few people with schizophrenia are in employment (Rosenheck et al. 2006).

Table 1.1: Symptoms of schizophrenia

Positive symptoms (that are not normal for the person):

- Hallucinations
- Delusions
- Thought disorder.

Negative symptoms (that the person doesn't usually experience):

- Poor motivation
- Social isolation
- Withdrawal.

Cognitive symptoms:

- Impaired attention and memory
- Difficulty with forward planning and problem solving.

Affective or mood symptoms:

- Signs of depression and/or anxiety.

Adapted from Andreasen (1995)

Epidemiology

Schizophrenia is not a common illness but it affects approximately one person in a hundred at some point in their lives (Saha et al. 2008). A meta-analysis of international studies of schizophrenia using pooled data found a prevalence estimate of 4.2 per 1000 (Saha et al. 2008).

Onset tends to be when people are in their teens to early twenties, and although schizophrenia is equally common in men and women, men tend to develop the illness when they are younger than women. This may be explained by the female hormone oestrogen having a protective effect against schizophrenia (Palmer et al. 2001).

Causes

Around 50 per cent of the cause of schizophrenia can be attributed to genetics (Tsuang et al. 2001). It occurs in 10 per cent of people who have a first-degree relative with the disorder, and is still more likely to develop in those who have second-degree relatives with the disease than in the general population. The identical twin of a person with schizophrenia has a 40–65 per cent chance of developing the disorder (Cardno & Gottesman 2000). Several genes are associated with an increased risk of schizophrenia (Harrison & Weinberger 2005).

Research has found that people with schizophrenia have higher rates of rare genetic mutations involving hundreds of different genes (Walsh et al. 2008). Other recent studies suggest that schizophrenia may result when a gene malfunctions that is needed to make important brain chemicals. This problem may affect the part of the brain involved in developing higher functioning skills (Huang *et al.* 2007).

Interactions between genes and the environment are necessary for schizophrenia to develop. Many environmental factors may be involved, such as exposure to viruses or malnutrition before birth, problems during birth, and other unknown psychosocial factors (Tsuang *et al.* 2001).

An imbalance in the complex, interrelated chemical reactions of the brain involving the neurotransmitters dopamine and glutamate, and possibly others, also plays a role in schizophrenia. Studies of brain tissue after death have revealed changes in the distribution or characteristics of brain cells (leading to faulty connections) that could have occurred before birth (Mueser & McGurk 2004). The problem may not manifest in a person until puberty when the brain undergoes major changes; these changes can then trigger psychotic symptoms.

In a study of 229 people with schizophrenia, the majority had prominent positive symptoms and a sudden onset of disease, with 69 per cent of the cases having a record of heavy cannabis abuse at least one year before onset of psychotic symptoms. The authors argue that the high number of cases of schizophrenia in this cohort, and the temporal link between cannabis abuse and schizophrenia, supports the hypothesis that cannabis abuse may be a risk factor for schizophrenia (Allebeck *et al.* 1993).

Early detection of schizophrenia

Making a diagnosis of schizophrenia requires psychotic symptoms to be present for at least a month (American Psychiatric Association 2013). Early detection and treatment is essential in order to ensure that persons are effectively treated as quickly as possible. Intervening early can improve the outcome of the illness and can reduce the risk of suicide (Melle *et al.* 2006). Schizophrenia often starts with increasing social isolation and deterioration in intellectual functioning (Andreasen 1995).

Diagnosis

The *Diagnostic and Statistical Manual of Mental Disorders* (5th edition; DSM-V) contains the recommended criteria for health professionals in the United Kingdom to use when making a diagnosis of schizophrenia and bipolar disorder (American Psychiatric Association 2013 – see Table 1.2).

Table 1.2: DSM-V diagnostic criteria for schizophrenia

Two or more of the following symptoms during a one-month period (or one of these if the delusions are bizarre or hallucinations are commentary style):

- Delusions
- Hallucinations
- Disorganised speech (e.g. incoherence or derailed thinking)
- Grossly disorganised or catatonic behaviour

- Negative symptoms (e.g. avolition (loss of ability to motivate, choose or resolve), lack of planning, emotional blunting or poverty of speech)
- Social or occupational dysfunction (disturbance in one or more major areas, such as work, self-care or interpersonal relationships)
- Continuous signs of disturbance for at least six months.

Criteria:

- Schizoaffective disorder and mood disorder with psychosis have been ruled out
- Substance misuse or a general medical condition have been excluded
- If autistic disorder or another pervasive developmental disorder is present, then schizophrenia can only be diagnosed if prominent delusions or hallucinations are present for at least one month.

■ ■ ■ Bipolar disorder

Bipolar disorder is a long-term condition characterised by episodes of elated mood (mania or hypomania) and depression (see Table 1.3). Making a diagnosis of bipolar disorder is challenging. Many people therefore experience long delays before being diagnosed with bipolar disorder, with an average of eight years from initial presentation to secondary care mental health services (Mantere et al. 2004). Substance use is extremely common, with both epidemiological and clinical studies showing rates ranging from 35 to 60 per cent (Grant et al. 2005), Frye et al. 2003, Chengappa 2000, Kessler et al. 1997, Feinman & Dunner 1996, Regier et al. 1990). Life expectancy is reduced in people with bipolar disorder due to the increased prevalence of CVD, respiratory disease and high rates of suicide (Colton & Manderscheid 2006).

Table 1.3: Symptoms of bipolar disorder

Depression:

- Feeling sad and hopeless, empty or worthless, guilty or despairing, pessimistic
- Lacking in energy
- Difficulty in concentrating and remembering things
- Loss of interest and enjoyment in everyday activities
- Self-doubt
- Problems with sleeping, and waking up early
- Suicidal thoughts.

Mania:

- Feeling extremely happy, elated or euphoric, full of energy, self-important, full of great new ideas and having important plans
- Talking quickly
- Being easily distracted, irritated or agitated
- Doing pleasurable things with distressing consequences, such as spending large amounts of money or having risky sexual encounters
- Not sleeping or eating.

Other:

- Psychosis may be present
- Some people self-harm as a distraction from mental pain and distress.

Adapted from American Psychiatric Association (2013)

Epidemiology

Bipolar disorder is divided into type I and type II. Type I involves episodes of mania, with or without episodes of depression. Type II is characterised by episodes of hypomania or elevated mood (but people are able to function) and depression (American Psychiatric Association 2013). The lifetime prevalence of bipolar I reported in European studies varies widely, from 0.1 to 2.4 per cent (Pini et al. 2005, ten Have et al. 2002, Szadoczky et al. 1998). An Australian study reported a lifetime prevalence of 2.5 per cent (Goldney et al. 2005). Estimates of the lifetime prevalence of bipolar II disorder also vary widely. Authors of European studies estimate between 0.2 and 2.0 per cent prevalence (Faravelli et al. 1990, Szadoczky et al. 1998).

Signs and symptoms of bipolar disorder

Mania

Manic symptoms include an elated mood accompanied by increased drive, over-activity and decreased need for sleep. The person thinks at speed and this is expressed in pressure of speech. To begin with, they may work more efficiently – until symptoms of poor concentration and distractibility occur. Some people experience extreme irritability. Common features include:

- Hallucinations and mood congruent delusions occur in 9 out of 10 people.
- Loss of social inhibitions and extravagant plans may result in grave consequences for an individual's professional life, social functioning and financial stability.
- Mania often results in such severe disruption of functioning that hospital admission is necessary, sometimes requiring compulsory detention.

Depression

The symptoms and the diagnostic criteria of depression in bipolar disorder are the same as those for unipolar depression: low mood; loss of interest and pleasure; reduced energy; poor concentration; disturbed sleep; a change in appetite; and low self-esteem and confidence (American Psychiatric Association 2013). Some individuals have ideas of guilt and hopelessness, and suicide may occur. Psychotic symptoms may feature in severe episodes and are typically mood congruent (American Psychiatric Association 2013).

In comparison to unipolar depression, bipolar depression is more likely to present with psychomotor retardation, melancholic symptoms such as a sense of worthlessness and psychosis and atypical features such as hypersomnia (Hardy & Gray 2012a). Bipolar depressive episodes are typically shorter than in unipolar depression. However, people presenting with depression directly following mania may be less likely to respond to treatment.

Mixed states

Some people with bipolar disorder can experience a mixed emotional state consisting of both mania and depression at the same time (American Psychiatric Association 2013); for example, racing thoughts during a manic episode.

Diagnosis

Das *et al.* (2005) report that bipolar disorder is associated with a high attendance rate in primary care, which provides an opportunity for detection. However, their study showed that little attention has been given to primary care patients who have current depression and past episodes of hypomania or mania, and the fact that their history may indicate bipolar disorder and a need for specialised treatment.

DSM-V criteria for a depressive episode

To meet the criteria for a major depressive episode, the person should have been experiencing at least five symptoms for at least two weeks. One of the symptoms has to be depressed mood or loss of interest or pleasure; there should also be distress or impairment in social or occupational functioning (American Psychiatric Association 2013).

DSM-V criteria for a manic episode

The DSM-V criteria for a manic episode are: a distinct period of abnormally and persistently elevated, expansive or irritable mood, lasting one week (or any duration if hospitalisation is necessary). During the period of mood disturbance, three or more symptoms should have persisted (four if the mood is only irritable) and have been present to a significant degree (American Psychiatric Association 2013).

Early intervention

Early intervention in people with bipolar disorder can be effective in improving long-term outcomes. Early intervention enables healthcare professionals to ensure that the person receives prescribed medication and adheres to an effective treatment regime. Many people with bipolar disorder never consult secondary care mental health services (ten Have *et al.* 2002).

What treatments are used in severe mental illness?

This chapter covers the treatments used in schizophrenia and bipolar disorder.

■ ■ ■ Schizophrenia

Schizophrenia requires treatment with antipsychotic medication to stabilise psychosis and prevent relapse of symptoms. Although many people with schizophrenia express a desire to stop their medication, good adherence is essential to ensure effective management of the illness and psychosocial recovery.

Antipsychotic medication

Antipsychotics reduce psychosis by diminishing abnormal transmission of dopamine. They do this by blocking the dopamine D2/3 receptor (not D1 or D4). Although several brain regions may be involved, it has been suggested that the ventral striatal regions may have a particularly critical role (Kapur et al. 2006).

Typical antipsychotics include chlorpromazine, haloperidol, pimozide and zuclopenthixol. They were first introduced in the 1950s. Although still commonly used, most people with schizophrenia are now treated with atypical antipsychotic drugs that started to be introduced in the early 1990s (Nasrallah 2003). Atypical antipsychotics include clozapine, olanzapine, quetiapine, risperidone and aripiprazole.

All antipsychotics (both typical and atypical) are equally clinically effective against the positive symptoms of schizophrenia. The older or typical drugs do not improve the negative symptoms associated with low levels of dopamine in the cortex (Van Rossum 1967). As might be predicted by their pharmacology, atypical medicines seem to be more effective in treating some of the negative and cognitive symptoms and may be more helpful in treating mood symptoms of schizophrenia (Darbàa et al. 2011). This is because they are also serotonin (5-HT) antagonists at the 5-HT2A receptor subtype; they therefore mitigate the negative signs and symptoms of schizophrenia by disinhibiting the dopamine system in the nigrostriatum and prefrontal cortex (Burns 2001).

Approximately one-fifth of people with schizophrenia will fail to respond to treatment with antipsychotic medication (typical or atypical) and are deemed to have treatment-resistant schizophrenia (Pantelis & Lambert 2003). These people should be treated with a drug called clozapine. This is a complex drug to use but very effective (Pantelis & Lambert 2003). In about 1 per cent of people it can cause agranulocytosis; consequently they will require regular blood monitoring and should be registered with a clozapine person-monitoring service (Atkin et al. 1996).

Side effects

Antipsychotic medicines can cause a number of side effects.

Extrapyramidal symptoms

Typical antipsychotics have diffuse effects, blocking dopamine receptors throughout the brain. As a result, they cause a range of dopamine-related side effects that include extrapyramidal symptoms (EPS). These include dystonia, akathisia and tardive dyskinesia. The newer atypical medicines have lower affinity for dopamine receptors and this results in less EPS (Worrel et al. 2000).

Other side effects

One study has shown that long-term treatment with antipsychotic drugs is associated with lower mortality, compared with no antipsychotic use (Tiihonen et al. 2009). However, some of the newer antipsychotic drugs have a greater tendency to cause physical problems (Nasrallah 2003). They can induce endocrine abnormalities (for example, diabetes and galactorrhoea), metabolic abnormalities (for instance, lipid abnormalities and weight gain) and cardiovascular side effects such as lengthening of the QT interval on electrocardiography (Holt & Peveler 2005, Nasrallah 2003, Thakore 2002). As people with schizophrenia often have a number of cardiovascular disease risk factors (such as smoking, poor diet and physical inactivity), it is these factors that are included in a lifestyle management programme rather than the choice of antipsychotic medication. These problems are discussed in more detail in Chapter 5.

Other types of treatment

Antipsychotic medication is the main treatment for schizophrenia. In addition, the authors of a meta-analysis have concluded that family intervention should be offered to people with schizophrenia who are in contact with carers, and that cognitive behavioural therapy (CBT) may be useful for those with treatment-resistant symptoms (Pilling et al. 2002). This is recognised by the authors of the government guidelines for schizophrenia (NICE 2014), who recommend offering:

● CBT to assist in promoting recovery in people with persisting positive and negative symptoms and for people in remission
● Family intervention to families of people with schizophrenia who live with or are in close contact with them (this may be particularly useful for families of those who have recently relapsed or are at risk of relapse or have persisting symptoms)
● Arts therapies to assist in promoting recovery, particularly in people with negative symptoms
● Peer support to help improve service user experience and quality of life.

■ ■ ■ Bipolar disorder

Medication is used in bipolar disorder to treat depression and mania, and to prevent depressive and manic symptoms from returning. Therefore, many people require treatment with more than one medication. The medications used to treat bipolar disorder include:

- **Antipsychotic medication**, as described earlier in this chapter
- **Valproate**
- **Lithium**
- **Lamotrigine**
- **Carbamazepine**
- **Selective serotonin reuptake inhibitors (SSRIs)**
- **Benzodiazepines**.

Valproate

Valproate (2-propylpentanoic acid) is an anticonvulsant drug used in the treatment of bipolar disorder (Fisher & Broderick 2003). It has a number of side effects, including change in appetite, constipation, diarrhoea, dizziness, drowsiness, hair loss, headache, indigestion, mild pain or redness at the injection site, nausea, stomach cramps or pain, trouble sleeping, vomiting, weakness and weight gain.

Lithium

Lithium is used for the prophylaxis of bipolar disorder (Cookson 2001). It is highly effective at preventing relapse (particularly manic episodes) and reducing the risk of suicide (Cipriani *et al.* 2005, Geddes *et al.* 2004). However, due to the risk of toxicity, lithium should only be started under specialist supervision, and thyroid function, creatinine and plasma lithium levels need to be monitored regularly (Geddes *et al.* 2004). Lithium can also cause weight gain.

Lamotrigine

Lamotrigine is an anticonvulsant used to prevent depressive episodes associated with bipolar disorder. Side effects include nausea, vomiting, diarrhoea, dry mouth, aggression, agitation, headache, drowsiness, dizziness, tremor, insomnia, ataxia, back pain, arthralgia, nystagmus, diplopia and blurred vision.

Carbamazepine

Carbamazepine is an anticonvulsant used for the prophylaxis of bipolar disorder (British National Formulary 2014). Side effects include dry mouth, nausea, vomiting, oedema, ataxia, dizziness, drowsiness, fatigue, headache, hyponatraemia, blood disorders, dermatitis and urticaria.

Selective Serotonin Reuptake Inhibitors (SSRIs)

SSRIs are anti-depressants that work by inhibiting pre-synaptic reuptake of the neurotransmitter serotonin (5-hydroxytryptamine, 5HT). This increases the availability of serotonin at synapses and enhances stimulation of postsynaptic neurones. The increased synaptic serotonin causes changes in receptor sensitivity, which helps to reduce depression. Side effects include headache, changes in sleep pattern, gastrointestinal function and sexual functioning. The use of SSRIs in bipolar disorder is controversial, as they can cause some individuals to rebound into mania (Goodwin 2009).

Benzodiazepines

Benzodiazepines are used as anxiolytics, sedatives, hypnotics, anticonvulsants and/or skeletal muscle relaxants. They are helpful for the treatment of behavioural disturbance or agitation in bipolar disorder. However, they should not be used in the long term because of the risk of dependence.

Acute or mixed episode

An acute manic or mixed episode of bipolar disorder may require treatment with a number of medications. Some people will also be admitted to hospital or receive care from a crisis or home treatment team. Goodwin (2009) explains which drugs to use in each phase:

● Antipsychotics to bring mania under control and treat any psychosis (alternative treatments are valporate, lithium and carbamazepine)

● Sleep problems and behavioural disturbances can be treated with PRN benzodiazepines

● Anti-depressant medication should be gradually stopped in people experiencing a manic episode of illness – in order to prevent further mania.

Psychological treatments are not effective in this phase of the illness.

Acute depressive episode

Goodwin (2009) describes how a person should be treated in this phase:

● SSRIs – but, to prevent a switch to mania, they can be co-prescribed with lithium, valporate or an antipsychotic. Then after 12 weeks, taper treatment off and stop.

● Lamotrigine may also be a potentially helpful treatment.

There is compelling evidence, from a number of randomised controlled trials, that quetiapine is effective in the treatment of bipolar depression (including any anxiety) and does not appear to switch people into mania (Calabrese et al. 2005).

Long-term treatment

Long-term treatment (for at least two years, following the first episode of illness) is required in bipolar disorder to prevent the recurrence of both the depressive and manic poles of the illness.

Psychological therapies

As an addition to medication, psychosocial treatments are helpful in providing support, education and guidance to people with bipolar disorder and their families (NICE 2006). Psychosocial interventions can lead to increased mood stability, fewer hospitalisations, and improved functioning in several areas (NICE 2006). Therapies that have been found to be helpful are described in Table 2.1 below.

Table 2.1: Psychological therapy

After an acute episode

Consider individual structured psychological interventions, such as CBT, in addition to prophylactic medication for people who are relatively stable, but may have mild to moderate affective symptoms. The therapy should normally be at least 16 sessions, over six to nine months, and:

• Include psychoeducation, the importance of a regular routine and concordance with medication

• Cover monitoring mood, detecting early warnings and providing strategies to prevent progression into full-blown episodes

• Enhance general coping strategies

• Be delivered by therapists who have experience of people with bipolar disorder.

Consider a focused family intervention if appropriate. This should last six to nine months, and cover psychoeducation, ways to improve communication and problem solving.

Psychosocial support

Consider offering befriending services to people who would benefit from additional social support, particularly those with chronic depressive symptoms. This should be in addition to pharmacological and psychological treatments, and should be by trained volunteers, providing at least weekly contact for between two and six months.

Adapted from NICE (2006)

Systems of the body that are commonly affected in people with severe mental illness

We have assumed that readers have previous knowledge of these systems of the body. This chapter has been included to serve as a reminder.

■■■ The respiratory system

The main parts of the respiratory system are the airways, the lungs and linked blood vessels, and the muscles that enable breathing.

There are two processes involved in respiration, external and internal:

● External respiration (breathing) is the taking of oxygen from the air and returning carbon dioxide to it.
● Internal (gaseous exchange): glucose or other small molecules are oxidised to produce energy. This requires oxygen and generates carbon dioxide.

External respiration occurs in the respiratory tract. This starts at the nose and mouth, and then extends from the neck into the thorax via the trachea. The trachea divides into the right and left bronchi, which enter the right and left lungs. (The right lung has three lobes and the left has two – it is smaller to allow room for the heart.) These bronchi further divide into smaller bronchi and bronchioles, which end in small air sacs called alveoli. Gaseous exchange occurs in the alveoli.

Each lung is surrounded by the pleura, a cavity filled with a thin layer of fluid and enclosed in the ribcage, confined below by the diaphragm and at the sides by the chest wall and the mediastinum. When the person breathes in, the ribcage expands; the pleural layers slide over each other and the pressure in the lung is decreased, so air is drawn in. When the person breathes out, the reverse happens; the ribcage collapses and air is expelled. The main element working in breathing is the diaphragm (a convex, domed layer of muscle). When it contracts, it flattens and increases the space above it. When the diaphragm relaxes, the abdominal contents push it up again. Between the ribs run two sets of intercostal muscles. The external intercostals run forward and downwards, and the internal intercostals run up and back. When the intercostal muscles contract, the ribs move up and out, which also increases the available space.

Internal respiration takes place in the lungs. Through the walls of the alveoli, oxygen from the air breathed in passes to the surrounding capillaries. The protein haemoglobin (which is present in red blood cells) helps move the oxygen from the alveoli to the blood. Carbon dioxide moves from the capillaries into the alveoli. The oxygenated blood from the lungs is carried through a network of capillaries to the pulmonary vein, which takes it to the left side of the heart. The left side of the heart pumps the blood to the rest of the body. There, the oxygen in the blood moves from blood vessels into the surrounding tissues. The pulmonary arteries carry deoxygenated blood from the heart to the lungs.

Breathing is controlled by the medulla oblongata and the pons in the brain. It is automatic but a person can consciously change their breathing rate. The breathing pattern can also be affected by emotions, activity, air quality and illness.

■■■ The reproductive system

The reproductive system is required for the continuation of the species. Both the male and the female contribute genetic material to create a new individual. The reproductive systems of both sexes mature during puberty. The ovaries of the female release eggs and the male's testes produce sperm. Reproduction occurs following sexual intercourse, when a sperm fuses with an egg (to form a foetus). This process is called fertilisation.

The female reproductive system

The female reproductive system contains a pair of ovaries. These organs are located in the female pelvis, on each side of the uterus. Each one is about the size and shape of an almond. They are components of both the reproductive and endocrine system (see p. 16). The ovaries produce eggs and the female hormones oestrogen and progesterone. These hormones affect the way breasts and body hair grow, as well as body shape, the menstrual cycle and pregnancy.

The uterus is the organ where the foetus develops. The endometrium (lining of the uterus) prepares for pregnancy each month by becoming thicker. During ovulation, a mature egg enters one of the paired fallopian tubes. If it is fertilised by a sperm, it will move on to the uterus to develop into a foetus. If fertilisation does not occur, the lining is discharged and menstruation occurs.

At the base of the uterus is the cervix, which widens to allow the birth of the baby. The vagina is a muscular tube that extends from the uterus to the outside of the body; it is part of the birth canal. During sexual intercourse, sperm is ejaculated here.

In pregnancy, the hormones oestrogen and progesterone influence the breasts and mammary glands to enlarge. Two days after birth, blood levels of these hormones drop, which stimulates the pituitary gland to release the hormone prolactin. Milk is then produced. The milk flows through openings in each nipple when suckled by the baby.

The male reproductive system

The male reproductive system is made up of the testes and penis. The testes are a pair of oval-shaped organs within the scrotal sac, which is located directly behind the penis and in front of the anus. Like the ovaries, the testes are components of both the reproductive and endocrine system. Their primary function is to produce sperm and to produce androgens (hormones that stimulate or control the development and maintenance of male characteristics), primarily testosterone.

Sperm cells mature and are stored in a tube called the epididymis. During ejaculation, they travel from the epididymis to the urethra (a tube that extends from the bladder to the tip of the penis) through another tube called the vas deferens. Sperm is mixed with other secretions to form seminal fluid (semen) before ejaculation.

The penis is the organ that transports the semen into the female vagina. It consists of the shaft, the glans and the foreskin. During sexual arousal, blood vessels in the tissue of the penis fill with blood, causing it to swell and become erect. It then becomes firm, longer and wider, enabling it to enter the female vagina.

■ ■ ■ The musculoskeletal system

The musculoskeletal system is made up of bones, muscles, joints, cartilage, tendons and ligaments.

Bones

The bones give the body shape and support by providing a framework. This protects the internal organs such as the heart, lungs and liver. Bones are categorised as being short, long, flat, irregular or sesamoid, according to their shape. For example, the carpals and tarsals are short; the humerus, tibia and femur are long; the scapula and sternum are flat; the vertebrae, and sacrum are irregularly shaped; and the patella is a sesamoid. Bones store salts and metabolic materials and serve as a site for the body's production of erythrocytes (red blood cells).

Muscles

Muscles can be divided into three categories: voluntary, involuntary and cardiac. Voluntary muscles allow for conscious movement of body parts, such as walking, waving or picking something up. Involuntary muscles are located within certain internal organs such as the stomach, intestine, bladder and blood vessels. Cardiac muscles are found within the heart, providing a constant pumping action.

Joints

Joints, with voluntary muscles, assist in the conscious movement of a body part. They are located where bones connect. They are constructed to allow movement (except for skull bones) and provide mechanical support.

Cartilage

Cartilage is a flexible connective tissue found in many areas in the body, including the joints between bones, the ribcage, the ear and the intervertebral discs. It is not as hard and rigid as bone but it is stiffer and less flexible than muscle.

Tendons

Tendons (also known as sinews) are tough bands of fibrous connective tissue made of collagen. They usually connect muscle to bone and are capable of withstanding tension. Tendons work with muscles to move bones.

Ligaments

Ligaments are formed of fibrous connective tissue made of collagen. They connect one bone to another bone to form a joint.

■ ■ ■ The endocrine system

The endocrine system's main purpose is regulating metabolism, growth and development, tissue function, sexual function, reproduction and sleep and mood. The endocrine system (*endo* meaning 'within' and *crinis* meaning 'secrete') is the collection of eight major glands that secrete different types of hormones: the pituitary gland, pineal gland, hypothalamus, thyroid gland, thymus, pancreas, adrenal glands and gonads (ovaries in females and testes in males). These glands are vascular and generally do not have ducts (unlike exocrine glands). They use intracellular vacuoles to store hormones. The hormones are released from the endocrine tissue into the bloodstream, where they travel to the target tissue to elicit a response. Some organs (such as the gonads, kidney, liver, and heart) have secondary endocrine functions. For example, the kidney secretes the hormones erythropoietin and renin.

Pituitary gland

The pituitary gland is located in the middle of the base of the brain, inferior to the hypothalamus. It is often called 'the master gland' because it directs other organs and endocrine glands to suppress or induce hormone production. Its functions include the production of growth hormone and hormones that act on other endocrine glands and the muscles and kidneys, endocrine function regulation and storage of hormones produced by the hypothalamus.

Pineal gland

The pineal gland is situated in the brain between the cerebral hemispheres, attached to the third ventricle. Melatonin is one of the hormones produced by this gland. Melatonin influences sexual development and sleep–wake cycles. The pineal gland connects the endocrine system with the nervous system by converting nerve signals from the sympathetic system of the peripheral nervous system into hormone signals.

Hypothalamus

The hypothalamus is located in the brain, inferior to the thalamus, posterior to the optic chiasm and bordered on the sides by the temporal lobes and optic tracts. It is the control centre for many autonomic functions of the peripheral nervous system, playing a vital role in maintaining homeostasis (temperature control, pH balance, water and electrolyte balance, blood pressure and respiration). The hypothalamus is part of the limbic system, which influences many of our emotions and motivations, particularly those related to survival. These include fear, anger, eating and sexual behaviour. Other functions include motor function control, the regulation of food and drink intake and the regulation of sleep.

Thyroid gland

The thyroid gland is located in the front of the neck, below the larynx, and consists of two lobes, one on each side of the trachea, connected by tissue called the isthmus. The thyroid tissue is made up of follicular cells and parafollicular cells. The follicular cells secrete iodine-containing hormones called thyroxine (T4) and triiodothyronine (T3). (Iodine is required to produce these hormones.) The follicular cells stimulate every tissue in the body to produce proteins and increase the amount of oxygen used by cells. The parafollicular cells secrete the hormone calcitonin. This works together with the parathyroid hormone to regulate calcium levels in the body. The levels of hormones secreted by the thyroid are controlled by the thyroid-stimulating hormone (TSH), produced in the pituitary gland, which is in turn controlled by the hypothalamus.

Thymus gland

The thymus gland is immediately beneath the breastbone, at the level of the heart. It is called thymus because its pyramid shape resembles that of a thyme leaf. It is made of two lobes that join in front of the trachea. The thymus plays an important part in a child's immune system. It grows larger until puberty and then begins to atrophy. The main thymus gland function is to produce and process lymphocytes (white blood cells or leukocytes) or T cells, which are the main element in the body's immune system. Another function of the thymus gland is to prevent the abnormal growth of cells that may lead to cancer.

Pancreas

The pancreas is an oblong, flattened gland, located deep in the abdomen and sandwiched between the stomach and the spine. It lies partially behind the stomach and in the curve of the duodenum. The pancreas has an exocrine component in addition to the endocrine function (acinar cells that produce enzymes to aid digestion). The endocrine cells are the islets of langerhans. They produce and secrete the hormones insulin and glucagon into the bloodstream. These hormones work together to maintain the right level of glucose in the blood.

Adrenal glands

The adrenal glands are triangle-shaped glands located on top of the kidneys. The outer part of the adrenal gland is called the cortex and produces the steroid hormones cortisol, aldosterone and testosterone. These have an effect on blood pressure and blood glucose levels, growth and some sexual characteristics. The inner part of the adrenal gland is called the medulla and produces adrenaline and noradrenaline, which regulate the body's 'fight or flight' response.

Ovaries and testes

The ovaries and testes are part of the endocrine system and are described in the reproductive system section (p. 14) above.

■ ■ ■ The cardiovascular system

The cardiovascular system is a network of organs and vessels responsible for the flow of blood, nutrients, oxygen and other gases, and hormones, to and from cells. The system is made up of the heart, circulatory loops and blood vessels.

The heart

The heart is located medial to the lungs, along the body's midline, in the thoracic region. About two-thirds of the heart is located on the left side of the body, as the bottom tip of the heart is turned to the left. The top of the heart (the heart's base) connects to the great blood vessels of the body (the aorta, vena cava, pulmonary trunk and pulmonary veins). Greater contractile force and heart rate lead to an increase in blood pressure.

Circulatory loops

There are two main circulatory loops in the body: the pulmonary circulation loop and the systemic circulation loop:

- The pulmonary circulation loop transports deoxygenated blood from the right side of the heart to the lungs, where the blood picks up oxygen and returns to the left side of the heart.
- The systemic circulation loop carries oxygenated blood from the left side of the heart to all the tissues of the body (except the heart and lungs). It also removes waste from body tissues and returns deoxygenated blood to the right side of the heart.

Blood vessels

Blood vessels allow blood to flow from the heart to every region of the body and back again. They contain a hollow area called the lumen, through which blood is able to flow. Around the lumen is the wall of the vessel. This is thin in capillaries and thick in arteries. The vessels are lined with a thin layer of simple squamous epithelium, known as the endothelium, which lines the entire circulatory system (called endocardium in the interior of the heart).

There are three major types of blood vessels: arteries, capillaries and veins. Blood vessels can increase blood pressure through vasoconstriction (a decrease in the diameter of an artery by contracting the smooth muscle in the arterial wall) and decrease it through vasodilatation (expansion of an artery as the smooth muscle in the arterial wall relaxes).

Functions of the cardiovascular system

There are three major functions of the cardiovascular system: transportation, protection and regulation of homeostasis.

Transportation

The blood delivers essential nutrients and oxygen, and removes wastes and carbon dioxide to be processed or removed from the body. The blood's liquid plasma transports hormones.

Protection

The blood contains a number of different blood cells that protect the body from infection and injury. The white blood cells clean up cellular debris and fight pathogens. The platelets and red blood cells form scabs to seal wounds and prevent pathogens from entering the body and liquids from leaking out. Antibodies are also carried in blood. They provide specific immunity to pathogens that the person has previously been exposed to, or has been vaccinated against.

Regulation

The cardiovascular system sustains homeostatic control of several internal conditions in three ways. Firstly, a stable body temperature is maintained by blood vessels controlling the blood flow to the surface of the skin. Secondly, the body's pH is balanced by the presence of bicarbonate ions, which act as a buffer solution. Lastly, the osmotic concentration of the body's cells is balanced by the albumins in blood plasma by maintaining an isotonic environment.

Common physical comorbidities in severe mental illness

There is evidence to show that people with SMI have an increased incidence of certain physical diseases. Oud and Meyboom-de Jong (2009) carried out a systematic review of 15 original research articles on somatic comorbidity in people suffering from psychotic disorders. They found that the prevalence of chronic physical illnesses in the SMI group was as high as 74 per cent.

In their comprehensive review of the literature, Leucht et al. (2007) highlighted the conditions for which there was good and very good evidence for increased risk in people with SMI (see Table 4.1).

Table 4.1: Prevalence of physical diseases in people with SMI

Disease category	Increased frequency
Bacterial infections and mycoses	Tuberculosis (+)
Viral diseases	HIV (++), hepatitis B/C (+)
Neoplasms	Obesity-related cancer (+)
Musculoskeletal diseases	Osteoporosis/decreased bone mineral density (+)
Stomatognathic diseases	Poor dental status (+)
Respiratory tract diseases	Impaired lung function (+)
Urological and male genital diseases	Sexual dysfunction (+)
Female genital diseases and pregnancy complications	Obstetric complications (++)
Cardiovascular diseases	Stroke, myocardial infarction, hypertension, other cardiac and vascular diseases (++)
Nutritional and metabolic diseases	Obesity (++), diabetes mellitus (+), metabolic syndrome (++), hyperlipidemia (++)

(++) Definitive evidence for increased risk (+) Probable evidence for increased risk

Adapted from Leucht et al. (2007)

■ ■ ■ The respiratory system

Tuberculosis

There are very few epidemiological studies on the association between schizophrenia and bacterial infections. Single studies from Japan (Ohta *et al.* 1988) and the United Kingdom (Baldwin 1979) found a higher incidence of tuberculosis (TB) among people with schizophrenia compared with the general population. Ohta *et al.* studied people living in a city and Baldwin looked at the statistical linkage between diseases using the Oxford Record Linkage Study from which in-patient data could be extracted.

Reports from Israel (Zeenreich *et al.* 1998) and Russia (Fisher *et al.* 1996) also indicated an increased prevalence of TB in psychiatric hospitals. As most of these studies were carried out in hospital settings, it could be argued that it is not the mental illness that is the risk factor for developing TB but the environment. This view is shared by Cavanaugh *et al.* (2012) who recently suggested that assisted living accommodation and residential homes (commonly housing people with SMI) may lack TB prevention infection control procedures. They report the example of one such facility for adults with mental illness in America. In 2008, 15 of the residents and three of the non-residents contracted tuberculosis. Residents were not routinely screened for medical problems.

Chronic obstructive pulmonary disease

The prevalence of chronic respiratory problems such as chronic obstructive pulmonary disease (COPD) is significantly higher in people with SMI (Himelhoch *et al.* 2004, Sokal *et al.* 2004, Chafetz *et al.* 2005, Carney *et al.* 2006, Copeland *et al.* 2007, Batki *et al.* 2009). This can be explained by the fact that approximately 50 per cent of people with SMI smoke, compared to 28 per cent in the general population (Vancampfort *et al.* 2013, Mitchell *et al.* 2011). A systematic review found that COPD was the most prevalent disease in this population (Oud & Meyboom-de Jong 2009). One study in the United Kingdom (Filik *et al.* 2006) found higher rates of lung function impairment in people with schizophrenia, compared to the general population.

■ ■ ■ The reproductive system

Human immunodeficiency virus (HIV)

There are many studies on the association between schizophrenia and HIV (Leucht *et al.* 2007). These show that the prevalence of HIV positivity in people with schizophrenia is generally higher than in the general population but is very variable. This may be because some studies were performed in high-risk areas (such as the east coast of the United States) while studies in other parts of the world (like Asia) showed lower HIV prevalence. Factors such as the high frequency of substance abuse, risky sexual behaviours and reduced knowledge of HIV-related issues could account for the higher prevalence. A study of 430 psychiatric outpatients in the United States

(Carey et al. 2004) found significant rates of risky sexual behaviour in people with SMI, particularly in those with mood disorders.

More recently, an American study examined 6,417,676 people who were without HIV in 2001 (Prince et al. 2012). The researchers compared the number of new diagnoses of HIV between 2002 and 2004 in people with SMI, a substance abuse disorder, and other psychiatric comorbidity. This showed that people with SMI did not have more new HIV/AIDS diagnoses than the general population but the likelihood of new diagnoses doubled if they also had a substance abuse disorder.

Hepatitis B/C

There has been little research carried out on hepatitis in psychiatric disorders, but studies from six different countries showed an increased prevalence of hepatitis in people with schizophrenia compared to the general population (Chaudhury et al. 1994, Cividini et al. 1997, Rosenburg et al. 2005, Said et al. 2001, Nakamura et al. 2004, Kalkan et al. 2005). A later study illustrated similar findings to those relating to HIV prevalence; 2.5 per cent of participants with SMI and a substance abuse disorder were infected with hepatitis, compared to 0.6 per cent of people without a substance abuse disorder (Rosenburg et al. 2005).

Sexual dysfunction

There are a number of relatively large studies that show sexual dysfunction to be more frequent in people with schizophrenia, compared to the rest of the population (Aizenberg et al. 1995, Smith et al. 2002, McDonald et al. 2003). The antipsychotic drugs prescribed to treat SMI are associated with sexual dysfunction as they can cause hyperprolactinaemia (Kasperek-Zimowska et al. 2008). The propensity to cause hyperprolactinaemia differs between antipsychotics as a result of differential dopamine D2 receptor-binding affinity and ability to cross the blood–brain barrier (Holt & Peveler 2011). This side effect has a significant negative impact on the person's satisfaction with treatment and their adherence to the medication (Hippisley-Cox et al. 2007).

Obstetric complications

There are many studies that demonstrate increased occurrence of obstetric complications among mothers with schizophrenia (De Hert et al. 2011). Most women with SMI cannot stop taking their medication, as this would interfere with their activities of daily living, especially taking care of a baby (Einarson & Boskovic 2009). However, so far, no definitive association has been found between the use of antipsychotics during pregnancy and an increased risk of birth defects or other adverse outcomes (Trixler et al. 2005, Einarson & Boskovic 2009). Therefore it may be the high rates of smoking, the use of illicit drugs and alcohol, and low socio-economic status that play a role in causing obstetric complications (Bennedsen 1998). There is an increased risk of psychosis following childbirth for women with bipolar disorder, which is not only a result of stopping mood-stabilising medication in pregnancy (Jones & Smith 2009).

■■■ The musculoskeletal system

Osteoporosis

People suffering from osteoporosis have decreased bone mineral density and are more likely to suffer from fractures (Halbreich & Palter 1996). Leucht et al. (2007) found 13 studies which consistently established that more people with schizophrenia had osteoporosis, compared to normal controls (Baastrup et al. 1980, Ataya et al. 1988, Delva et al. 1989, Halbreich et al. 1995, Keely et al. 1997, Bergemann et al. 2001, Bilici et al. 2002, Zhang-Wong & Seeman 2002, Abraham et al. 2003, Liu-Seifert et al. 2004, Meaney et al. 2004, Hummer et al. 2005, Kishimoto et al. 2005, O'Keane & Meaney 2005). Most of the studies examined had very small samples, the smallest and largest cohorts being 10 and 402 respectively. Despite this knowledge, there is evidence that people with schizophrenia receive less care for their osteoporosis than age-matched controls (Bishop et al. 2004).

Reduced bone mineral density can be caused by a sedentary lifestyle, lack of exercise, smoking, alcohol and drug abuse, dietary and vitamin deficiencies, decreased exposure to sunshine and polydipsia inducing electrolyte imbalance. These behaviours are frequently observed in people with schizophrenia (Halbreich & Palter 1996). Additionally, many antipsychotic drugs increase prolactin levels, which can cause osteoporosis (Holt & Peveler 2011).

A more recent meta-analysis (De Hert et al. 2011) has found further studies that confirm the increased prevalence of osteoporosis in people with mental illness, particularly those taking antipsychotics. However, they report that data describing the epidemiology of osteoporotic fracture and antipsychotics in people with SMI are limited and there are some conflicting results.

■■■ The endocrine and cardiovascular system

Cardiovascular disease

The most common cause of premature death in people with SMI is cardiovascular disease (CVD) (Hennekens et al. 2005). We describe this in detail in Chapter 5.

■■■ Various systems

Cancer

Studies relating to cancer and people with schizophrenia have had conflicting findings. Some have established that there is actually a decreased risk of cancer in this population (Barak et al. 2005, Dalton et al. 2005, Goldacre et al. 2005, Grinshpoon et al. 2005, Dalton et al. 2004, Lichtermann et al. 2001, Dalton et al. 2003, Cohen et al. 2001, Lawrence et al. 2000, Mortensen 1994, Gulbinat et al. 1992, Mortensen 1992, Mortensen 1989, Dupont et al. 1986, Nakane et al. 1986, Driscoli et al. 1978). The authors of these studies speculated that genetic factors that may lead to schizophrenia could protect the person from cancer. Other theories are that certain antipsychotic drugs may prevent tumours growing (Driscoli *et al.* 1978), or frequent admissions to hospital that provide good medical care and less exposure to urban air pollutants may be protective (Mortensen 1989, Grinshpoon *et al.* 2005, Goldacre *et al.* 2005, Dalton *et al.* 2003).

In contrast, a large study carried out in Finland found an increased cancer risk in people with schizophrenia (Lichtermann *et al.* 2001). The results are also contradictory when examining studies looking at specific cancer sites. For example, some studies show decreased risks of lung cancer in people with schizophrenia (Mortensen 1989, 1994) while others show increased risks (Lichtermann *et al.* 2001, Grinshpoon *et al.* 2005). Prostate cancer is an exception; the studies consistently found this to be rarer in the schizophrenia population than the general one (Barak *et al.* 2005, Dalton *et al.* 2005, Goldacre *et al.* 2005, Grinshpoon *et al.* 2005, Lichtermann *et al.* 2004, Lawrence *et al.* 2000, Mortensen 1992, Dupont *et al.* 1986).

More recently, in a cohort analysis within a large UK primary care database, the incidence of colorectal, breast and lung cancer, and of all common cancers, did not differ significantly in people with SMI, including schizophrenia, when compared with people without SMI (Osborn *et al.* 2013). It is worth noting that people with SMI are less likely to be screened for cancer. For example, a number of studies have shown that, in comparison to the general population, women with schizophrenia were less likely to have received a mammogram in the last two years than women of the same age in the general population (Chochinov 2009, Carney, Jones & Woolson 2006, Wernenke *et al.* 2006, Druss *et al.* 2002).

Turning from incidence of cancer to mortality from cancer, one study has shown that having SMI does not increase the risk of death from the seven most common cancers in the UK (Osborn *et al.* 2007).

Poor dental status

There are a number of studies that highlight the poor dental status of people with schizophrenia (Thomas *et al.* 1996, Velasco *et al.* 1997, Kenkre & Spadigam 2000, Lewis *et al.* 2001, McCreadie *et al.* 2004, Tang *et al.* 2004, Velasco-Ortega *et al.* 2005). Caries, gingivitis and periodontal disease may be caused by poor diet, neglecting oral hygiene and smoking. All these behaviours are common in people with schizophrenia (Frielander & Marder 2002). In addition, antipsychotics, anti-depressants and mood stabilisers can result in reduced saliva flow, which causes additional risk (Frielander & Marder 2002).

Cardiovascular disease in people with severe mental illness

Many risk factors for cardiovascular disease (CVD) are significantly increased in people with SMI (Osborn *et al.* 2006). They have a higher risk of developing metabolic syndrome (prevalence of 36 per cent) and there is an increased prevalence of diabetes mellitus (9–14 per cent) than among the general population (Holt & Peveler 2010, Oud & Meyboom-de Jong 2009).

The term CVD is mainly used to describe disorders affecting the heart and/or the arteries and veins that are associated with atherosclerosis (the build-up of fatty deposits and debris inside blood vessels). Coronary heart disease (CHD) and peripheral artery disease are long-term conditions but acute types of CVD (such as myocardial infarction and stroke) can occur suddenly, when a vessel supplying blood to the heart or brain becomes blocked or bursts.

It is the combination of lifestyle factors (McCreadie 2003), poorer physical healthcare (Thornicroft 2011) and the side effects of antipsychotic medication (De Hert *et al.* 2009) that result in the high incidence of CVD in people with SMI.

Family history and ageing are the strongest risk factors for developing CVD. The most important behavioural risk factors for CVD are unhealthy diet, physical inactivity and tobacco use, which together cause about 80 per cent of CHD and stroke (WHO 2011). The effects of these unhealthy behaviours can contribute to metabolic risk factors such as raised blood pressure, raised blood glucose and cholesterol, and obesity. Public health initiatives therefore focus on protecting against the development of CVD by encouraging people to follow a healthy diet, avoid smoking, exercise regularly, and maintain blood pressure, blood glucose and cholesterol within recommended limits. Underlying determinants of CVD may include poverty, stress and hereditary factors (WHO 2011), and the risk factors for CVD can be divided into unmodifiable and modifiable types.

■ ■ ■ Risk factors that cannot be modified

Risk factors that cannot be modified are those that a person cannot change, such as age, gender, ethnicity and genetics.

Age and gender

In the general population, the incidence of CVD increases with age (World Heart Federation 2012). CVD is more common in males than females up to the age of 65, when the incidence equalises across the genders (World Heart Federation 2012). Men aged 35 to 44 years are more than six times more likely to die from CVD than their female counterparts of the same age, although mortality due to CVD equalises in men and women over 75 years of age (Mercuro et al. 2010). In comparison, in a study of 46,163 people with SMI (Osborn et al. 2007), risk of death from CHD was increased between the ages of 18 and 75 years but did not increase further over the age of 75. The study also revealed that risk of stroke rose in people with SMI aged 18–49 years, but this increased risk disappeared in people aged over 50 years (Osborn et al. 2007).

Ethnicity

Risk factors vary significantly by ethnic group; for example, atherosclerotic disease and CHD are relatively rare in people of Afro-Caribbean extraction (Lip et al. 2007). Despite this group having an increased risk of glucose intolerance, very low-density lipoprotein (VLDL), small dense LDL, and lower triglyceride concentrations than in Europeans, the latter does not increase to the same extent in the presence of glucose intolerance (Chaturvedi et al. 1994).

In contrast, the prevalence rates of CVD in South Asians are at epidemic proportions (Lip et al. 2007). Risk factors such as smoking, blood pressure, obesity and cholesterol vary between subgroups of South Asians. Some levels are equivalent to, or lower than, a comparable European population; however, levels of glucose intolerance, central obesity, fasting triglyceride and insulin are uniformly elevated in comparison (McKeigue et al. 1991).

Family history

Individuals with a family history of CVD are at greater risk of an early CVD event (Williams et al. 2001). A positive family history means having a father diagnosed with CVD at less than 55 years of age or a mother diagnosed younger than 65 years of age (Wood et al. 1998).

■ ■ ■ Risk factors that can be modified

Modifiable risk factors are those that can be changed, such as obesity, dyslipidaemia, blood pressure and diabetes management, stress and poor lifestyle choices (physical activity, smoking, diet, alcohol intake – discussed in Chapter 6).

Several antipsychotic drugs, particularly the atypicals such as clozapine and olanzapine, appear to contribute to cardiometabolic risk. In individuals maintained on some of these antipsychotics, rates of metabolic syndrome and diabetes (or prediabetes) can exceed 50 per cent (Manu et al. 2012). In contrast, a number of studies found that the rate of metabolic syndrome is 10 per cent in persons with schizophrenia who are untreated (Manu et al. 2012, Chiu et al. 2010). This disparity could be due to the difference in severity of the SMI rather than the medication.

Obesity

There is strong evidence of an association between obesity and atherosclerosis, high blood pressure, high total blood cholesterol and type 2 diabetes (Wilson *et al.* 2002). This is due to an altered metabolic profile, and a variety of adaptations/alterations in cardiac structure and function as adipose tissue accumulates in excess amounts (Poirier 2006).

Some antipsychotic medication can cause weight gain (Allison & Casey 2001). One study concluded that histamine receptor blockade was the primary cause of antipsychotic-induced weight gain and diabetes mellitus (Matsui-Sakata *et al.* 2005). However, Holt and Peveler (2009) argue that it is too simplistic to ascribe all obesity in people with SMI to their drug treatment. They suggest that the development of obesity in SMI results from the complex interaction of the genotype and environment of the person with mental illness, the mental illness itself and antipsychotic medication.

Two recent meta-analyses of people with schizophrenia and bipolar disorder who were systematically monitored found approximately half were obese (Vancampfort *et al.* 2013, Mitchell *et al.* 2011).

Dyslipidaemia

The two major lipids (or fat chemicals) in the blood are cholesterol and triglyceride. As they are both insoluble, they are transported in the blood by lipoprotein structures: low-density lipoproteins (LDLs), known as 'bad' cholesterol; and high-density lipoproteins (HDLs), known as 'good' cholesterol. Dyslipidaemia is an abnormally high concentration of lipids or lipoproteins in the blood (it may also refer to abnormally low concentrations of HDL cholesterol) and is a risk factor for CVD. For example, a prospective cohort study of 7,587 women and 6,394 men showed that elevated triglyceride levels were associated with increased risk of heart disease and death (Nordestgaard *et al.* 2007).

A primary care study showed that patients with SMI had significantly lower HDL-cholesterol levels and higher total cholesterol to HDL-cholesterol ratio (Osborn *et al.* 2006). Two recent meta-analyses of people with SMI found that two in five had hypertriglyceridemia (Vancampfort *et al.* 2013, Mitchell *et al.* 2011).

Blood pressure

Persistently high blood pressure increases the risk of myocardial infarction and stroke (NICE 2011). The two most recent meta-analyses showed that two in five people with SMI had hypertension (Vancampfort *et al.* 2013, Mitchell *et al.* 2011). A study of 800 people with SMI in the UK found that 34 per cent were hypertensive (Eldridge *et al.* 2011). But in comparison, a UK survey of the general population showed that 32 per cent of men and 27 per cent of women aged over 35 were hypertensive (Health and Social Care information Centre 2010). Other studies have found little overall difference in the blood pressure of people with SMI compared with the general population (Osborn *et al.* 2006, Leucht *et al.* 2007). This may be due to the hypotensive effect of antipsychotic medication (Guggar 2011).

Diabetes

CVD is the main cause of death in people with diabetes, accounting for 50 per cent of all diabetes-related mortality and a high proportion of diabetes-related disability (Morrish et al. 2001). Diabetes occurs in 15 per cent of people with schizophrenia (Holt and Peveler 2005) compared with 5 per cent of the general population (Bushe and Holt 2004). More recent meta-analyses of people with SMI found one in three having metabolic syndrome, diabetes or prediabetes (Vancampfort et al. 2013, Mitchell et al. 2011). Risk factors include a family history of diabetes, physical inactivity, poor diet, smoking and the metabolic effects of antipsychotic medication (Gough & Peveler 2004). People with diabetes are three times more likely to suffer from depression (Goldney et al. 2004) and/or anxiety symptoms (Grigsby et al. 2002). This in turn further increases their risk of CVD due to poor self-management of their condition (Williams & Pickup 2004).

Psychosocial stress

There is increasing evidence to support the hypothesis that psychosocial stress is an important risk factor for CVD (Bairey Merz et al. 2002). People with schizophrenia have an impaired ability to adapt to stress (Kudoh et al. 1999).

Problematic behaviours affecting health in people with severe mental illness

In this chapter, the health behaviours that may be problematic in the SMI population are discussed. These involve physical activity, diet, alcohol intake, smoking, drug use, sexual behaviour, attitudes to health and adherence to treatment.

Physical activity

Regular physical activity decreases the risk of death from cardiovascular disesase (CVD) in general and death from coronary heart disease (CHD) in particular (Kesaniemi *et al.* 2001). Regular physical activity prevents or delays the development of high blood pressure and reduces blood pressure in people with hypertension (Fagard 1999). Exercise can also lower blood cholesterol levels and help with weight loss (Kantor *et al.* 1987). Low levels of exercise are common among people with SMI (Brown *et al.* 1999). This may be due to the symptoms of their condition (such as poor motivation) and/or the sedative effects of antipsychotic medication.

Eating

Diet affects blood cholesterol levels, body weight, blood pressure and blood glucose levels (Parikh *et al.* 2005). Studies have shown that the diets of people with SMI tend to be poor, for example lacking in fruit and vegetables (McCreadie *et al.* 2005), high in fat, salt and carbohydrates (Henderson *et al.* 2006) and low in nutritional content (Peet 2004).

Alcohol intake

Consumption of 1–2 units of alcohol a day is associated with a reduced risk of cardiovascular disease (Rimm *et al.* 1991, Marmota 1983). Government guidelines in the United Kingdom presently recommend a daily limit of 2–3 units (e.g. 175ml of ABV 13 per cent wine is a standard glass of wine and is 2.3 units) for women and 3–4 units for men (e.g. 1 pint of ABV 5.2 per cent beer is 3.1 units) (Drinkaware 2011).

Excessive alcohol intake is associated with increased all-cause mortality (Vogel 2002). There is little recent evidence regarding alcohol and people with SMI. The National Psychiatric Morbidity Survey in England found that 16 per cent of people with schizophrenia were drinking over the recommended weekly limits, for that time, of 21 units of alcohol for men and 14 units of alcohol for women (Meltzer et al. 1996). A population survey found high alcohol use in people with bipolar disorder (Kessler et al. 1997).

Smoking

Smoking rates are high in people with SMI. Two meta-analyses of people with SMI found that approximately half smoked (Vancampfort et al. 2013, Mitchell et al. 2011). More recently, a study showed the same results, with approximately 50 per cent of people with SMI smoking, compared with 28 per cent of the general population (Osborn et al. 2013).

People with SMI have reported an improvement in their symptoms when using smoking to self-medicate (Johnson et al. 2010). This may be due to an increased dopamine release in the pre-frontal cortex that alleviates positive and negative symptoms (Lavin et al. 1996). There may also be a reduction in the side effects of antipsychotic medication because of the enhanced metabolism of these drugs in smokers (Jeste et al. 1996).

Drug use

In the largest assessment of substance use among individuals with SMI to date, it was found that they had increased use of recreational drugs, compared to the general population (Hartz et al. 2014). In addition, the protective factors associated with belonging to certain racial or ethnic groups, or being female, did not appear to exist in these participants. These findings indicate that the rates of substance use in people with severe psychosis may be underestimated. There is a need for further research to find out more about the association between substance use and people with SMI so that both conditions can be treated successfully.

Sexual behaviour

Several studies have examined possible reasons why people with SMI may be at higher risk for HIV and other sexually transmitted infections (Gordon et al. 1999). These include: intravenous drug use; selling or swapping sex for cash or drugs; poor decision-making about safe sex (i.e. not insisting on condom use); the increased likelihood of having sex with someone who is injecting drugs (due to intoxication); hypersexuality; and vulnerability to coercion for sex (Gray et al. 2002, Cournos et al. 1994).

Awareness about HIV and sexual health risks is poor in SMI patients. For example, Kalichman et al. (1994) tested knowledge about HIV in 95 psychiatric outpatients (82 per cent had schizophrenia) and found that 37 per cent believed that showering after sex would prevent HIV infection, and a quarter thought that a person must have multiple sexual partners to get the virus. Some mental health professionals avoid talking to patients about sex. This does them a disservice, as they are an at-risk population and require appropriate interventions.

Attitudes to health

People with SMI experience more physical disease than the general population; yet they are less likely to pay attention to their lifestyle and physical health needs (Buhagiar *et al.* 2011). As lack of motivation is one of the symptoms of SMI, this may be an explanation. However, a poor understanding of the consequences of unhealthy behaviour may also be a factor.

Adherence to treatment

Maintenance treatment with antipsychotic medication is effective in preventing relapse in severe mental illness (Leucht *et al.* 2012) but requires patients to adhere to their treatment. As in other long-term conditions, around 50 per cent of patients with schizophrenia do not adhere to their medication regime (Lacro *et al.* 2002).

Non-adherence is associated with an increased risk of relapse, hospital admission and having persistent psychotic symptoms (Morken *et al.* 2008). Factors consistently associated with non-adherence include poor insight, negative treatment/illness beliefs, past non-adherence, and a poorer therapeutic relationship (Lacro *et al.* 2002). Effective interventions may include brief psychological intervention such as adherence (also known as compliance) therapy (AT; Schulz *et al.* 2013) and behavioural (Velligan *et al.* 2008) and financial incentive programmes (Priebe *et al.* 2013).

How to use the Health Improvement Profile (physical health check tool)

The Health Improvement Profile (HIP) is an evidence-derived physical health check tool specifically designed for people with severe mental illness (SMI). It can be defined as a physical health risk assessment. The tool was developed to support clinicians in identifying physical health problems and then guide them towards evidence-based interventions to address them. Cardiovascular disease (CVD) is highly prevalent and a major killer but there are other health issues and behaviours that also need to be tackled. The HIP addresses all the physical health problems that are more common in people with SMI. For instance, dental health is particularly poor in this patient group but is often overlooked.

When developing the HIP, two important factors had to be considered. Firstly, it needed to fit onto one side of A4, as it was felt that any questionnaire extending over two or more pages would be less likely to be completed by busy clinicians. Secondly, it had to offer a resource for practitioners who might be experienced in dealing with a patient's mental health issues but less experienced in addressing their physical health problems.

The male and female versions of the HIP are slightly different (for obvious reasons); both have 27 items, which are shown in Table 7.1. A copy of both versions of the HIP can be found at the back of this book. The HIP is copyright free but it would be helpful if you would let the authors know if you are planning to use the tool in practice. You can request the HIP through this website: http://physicalsmi.webeden.co.uk/

Although the objective of getting the HIP onto one side of A4 was achieved, the text is very dense. In practice, many clinicians therefore find it easier to print it on A3 paper.

The HIP should be completed once a year for every person with SMI; the National Institute for Health and Care Excellence (NICE) agree with this, and also recommend annual health checks. Who is responsible (primary care or secondary care) for doing health checks has been the subject of considerable (and trying) debate for well over a decade now. NICE suggests that GPs should be primarily responsible for doing health checks for people with SMI and they are financially rewarded (through their contract with the NHS) to do this work.

Table 7.1: HIP items

HIP item	Male	Female
Measurements		
Body mass index	Yes	Yes
Waist circumference	Yes	Yes
Pulse	Yes	Yes
Blood pressure	Yes	Yes
Temperature	Yes	Yes
Blood tests		
Liver function	Yes	Yes
Lipids	Yes	Yes
Glucose	Yes	Yes
Screening		
Prostate and testicles	Yes	No
Cervical cytology	No	Yes
Teeth	Yes	Yes
Eyes	Yes	Yes
Feet	Yes	Yes
Breast	Yes	Yes
Menstrual cycle	No	Yes
Urine	Yes	Yes
Bowels	Yes	Yes
Lifestyle		
Sleep	Yes	Yes
Smoking status	Yes	Yes
Exercise	Yes	Yes
Alcohol	Yes	Yes
Diet: literacy	Yes	Yes
Diet: function	Yes	Yes
Fluid intake	Yes	Yes
Caffeine intake	Yes	Yes
Cannabis use	Yes	Yes
Safe sex	Yes	Yes
Sexual satisfaction	Yes	Yes

The average GP practice, with 5,000 registered patients, will only have 50 with SMI. It is therefore not surprising that getting health checks done for this group is often not seen as a priority. Despite years of debate, research and policy writing, only a minority of people with SMI will have had a comprehensive health check each year, and those who have had one are unlikely to have a care plan that addresses the problems identified. By carrying out these health checks, healthcare practitioners working in secondary or social care would therefore be providing a much-needed service.

At the top of the HIP, there is space to record the person's age, ethnicity, weight, height and the date of HIP completion. The main HIP document is divided into seven columns. The first lists the parameter that is being assessed (e.g. BMI), and the second is a column to record the observed score (e.g. blood pressure = 152/95). The third column lists the normal range (e.g. pulse 60–100 beats per minute. The fourth column provides a box to tick if the observed score is within the normal range. The ticks in this column are described as green, suggesting that for this parameter the person is comparatively healthy. Abnormal ranges (e.g. no exercise taken) are set out in the sixth column. The sixth is a tick box indicating that the parameter is in the red and therefore unhealthy. The final column lists recommended action for parameters ticked red (e.g. refer to GP or specialist practice nurse).

A copy of the completed HIP should be given to the person, entered into their notes and sent to the GP. In studies where health checks have been carried out, it has been found that nurses take about 30–40 minutes to complete the HIP and typically people with SMI have nine red items (White 2010). Feedback from patients and professionals has always been very positive.

■■■ The HIP – item by item

Screening			
Item 1 Body mass index (BMI)	*Score*	*Green* 18.50–24.99	*Red* < 18.50 or ≥ 25.00

Rationale

Evidence suggests that excess weight gain can be two to three times more prevalent in people with schizophrenia than in the general population (Allison & Casey 2001). The BMI is a simple index used to determine whether an individual is underweight, overweight or obese (WHO 2006). The BMI is defined as the weight divided by the square of the height. For example, a person who weighs 70kg and has a height of 1.75m will have a BMI of 22.9. A BMI calculator can be found at: http://www.nhs.uk/Tools/Pages/Healthyweightcalculator.aspx

Although BMI values are the same for both sexes, they may not be accurate in people who are athletes or who weight-train, in pregnant or breastfeeding women, or those over the age of 60. Ethnicity should also be considered, particularly in people of South Asian origin (overweight varies from BMI > 23; obesity from BMI > 25).

Recommended action

Dietary advice should be offered to everyone to prevent weight gain (unless they are underweight). Guidance about weight loss should be offered to people with:

- A BMI ≥ 28
- Any degree of high BMI coinciding with diabetes or other serious diseases.

People who are underweight (BMI < 18.50) should be referred to their GP for investigation.

Item 2 Waist circumference	Score	Green < 80cm (female) < 94 cm (male)	Red ≥ 80cm (female) ≥ 94 cm (male)

Rationale

People who carry their excess fat centrally (within the abdominal cavity) are more likely to suffer the consequences of being overweight. Waist circumference correlates with visceral adipose tissue, plasma lipids, lipoproteins and insulin levels in adults (Taylor et al. 1998).

Recommended action

Measure waist circumference (ensure that a tape of adequate length is available). The correct position for measuring waist circumference is midway between the bottom of the ribcage and the uppermost border of the right iliac crest. The tape should be placed around the abdomen at this midway point and a reading taken when the tape is snug but does not compress the skin. In practice, it may be difficult in very overweight people to accurately palpate those bony landmarks, in which case placing the tape at the level of the belly button is recommended (National Obesity Forum 2011). For women with waist circumference ≥ 80 cm and men with waist circumference ≥ 94 cm (Barnett et al. 2007):

- Offer support and information on diet (e.g. meal planning) and exercise
- Consider referral to a local weight/exercise management programme
- Consider medication review.

Item 3 Pulse rate	Score	Green 60–100bpm	Red < 60bpm / > 100bpm

Rationale

Most antipsychotic medications have the potential for lengthening of the QT interval (prolonged: in males > 450ms, in females > 470ms [Committee for Proprietary Medicinal Products 1997]). Therefore, cardiac safety should be a routine part of clinical care in people taking antipsychotic medication; a preventive strategy is valuable even if the absolute risk of serious cardiac events is low (Abdelmawla & Mitchell 2006). There is evidence that many typical antipsychotics increase the risk of ventricular arrhythmias and cardiac arrest (Ray et al. 2001, Liperoti et al. 2005), and there is an association between many atypical antipsychotic drugs and the occurrence of unexplained sudden death (Abdelmawla & Mitchell, 2006).

Carrying out an ECG also allows the opportunity to look for other possible problems such as gynaecomastia, hygiene neglect and rashes.

Recommended action

Check pulse annually. If raised, perform an ECG. Consider an ECG for all individuals taking antipsychotics. The British National Formulary (BNF) recommends that an ECG should be performed on: those taking pimozide, sertinol and clozapine; those who have been prescribed antipsychotics over the BNF limits; those with specific cardiovascular risk; those with a personal history of cardiovascular disease; and anyone admitted as an inpatient.

People with an abnormal ECG may be referred to a cardiologist or to the original prescriber for review of their treatment as appropriate.

Item 4 Blood pressure	Score	Green < 140/90*	Red ≥ 140/90

Rationale

People with SMI are at higher risk of developing high blood pressure than the general population. The British Hypertension Society Guideline cites evidence that suboptimal blood pressure control leaves people at an unacceptably high risk of cardiovascular complications and death, particularly from coronary heart disease (CHD) but also from stroke (Williams *et al.* 2004). Interventions actively combining exercise and diet have demonstrated a reduction of both systolic and diastolic blood pressure by only 4–5mmHg (NICE 2011). Therefore blood pressure lowering medication is often required.

Recommended action

All people with SMI should be offered information on weight loss (if overweight), exercise, improved diet, reduction in alcohol and salt intake, and assistance with stopping smoking.

People with blood pressure > 140/90mmHg without a diagnosis of hypertension should be referred to the GP for ambulatory blood pressure monitoring (ABPM) or home blood pressure monitoring (HBPM) to confirm the diagnosis of hypertension (NICE 2011).

*People with another long-term condition, such as diabetes or stroke, may have a lower target for their blood pressure. This should be discussed with the practice nurse or GP.

Item 5 Temperature	Score	Green 36–37.5°C	Red < 36 ≥ 37.5°C

Rationale

A raised temperature maybe caused by infection, heat stroke, alcohol withdrawal, anticholinergic drugs, allergic drug reaction and agonist drugs (Dougherty & Lister 2004).

Neuroleptic malignant syndrome is a rare but potentially life-threatening individual reaction to neuroleptic drugs. It causes fever, muscular rigidity, altered mental status and autonomic dysfunction. It is usually associated with potent neuroleptics, such as haloperidol and fluphenazine. The underlying pathological abnormality is thought to be central D2 receptor blockade or dopamine depletion in the hypothalamus and nigrostriatal/spinal pathways. This leads to an elevated temperature set point, impairment of normal thermal homeostasis and extrapyramidally induced muscle rigidity (Patient UK 2006).

Recommended action

- Look for signs of infection and treat as appropriate.
- Ask about alcohol withdrawal.
- Check drug use.
- For abnormally high temperatures with fluctuating blood pressure and/or dystonia, consider neuroleptic malignant syndrome and refer urgently to medics.

Blood tests			
Item 6 Liver function tests (LFTs)	Score	Green In last 3 months*	Red More than 3 months*

Rationale

Antipsychotic medication can result in abnormal LFTs (Garcia-Unzueta *et al.* 2003).
Hepatic disease should be detected early to prevent further serious complications.

Recommended action

- Check LFTs every three months in people who have a newly prescribed or increased dose of antipsychotic.
- *Check LFTs every 12 months in people who are stable and have had no change in medication.
- If tests are abnormal, refer to the GP.

Item 7 Lipid levels	Score	Green TC < 5.1mmol/L LDL–C < 4.1mmol/L HDL–C >1.3mmol/L TG < 2.2mmol/L2	Red More than 3 months since last check if previous reading abnormal

Rationale

Dyslipidaemia is a key component of the metabolic syndrome and a precursor for CVD.

Recommended action

- Follow the national guidance (NICE 2014).

- Check cholesterol levels annually and lipid profile if cholesterol is raised. Offer support and information on diet (e.g. meal planning) and exercise.

Primary prevention

- Before starting lipid modification therapy for the primary prevention of CVD, take at least I lipid sample to measure a full lipid profile. A fasting sample is not needed.
- Offer atorvastatin 20 mg for the primary prevention of CVD to people who have a 10% or greater 10-year risk of developing CVD. Estimate the level of risk using the QRISK2 assessment tool.

Abnormal levels (secondary prevention)

- Start statin treatment with atorvastatin 80 mg. Use a lower dose of atorvastatin if any of the following apply: potential drug interactions; high risk of adverse effects; patient preference.
- Measure total cholesterol, HDL cholesterol and non-HDL cholesterol in all people who have been started on high-intensity statin treatment at 3 months of treatment and aim for a greater than 40% reduction in non-HDL cholesterol. If a greater than 40% reduction in non-HDL cholesterol is not achieved: discuss adherence and timing of dose; optimise adherence to diet and lifestyle measures; consider increasing dose if started on less than atorvastatin 80 mg and the person is judged to be at higher risk because of comorbidities, risk score or using clinical judgement.

Item 8	Score	Green	Red
Glucose		< 6.0 mmol/L	≥ 6.0 mmol/L
HbAIc		< 48 mmol/mol	≥ 48mmol/mol
		(Between 48 and 58 if patient has diabetes)	(Between 48 and 58 if patient has diabetes)

Rationale

Diabetes occurs in 15 per cent of people with schizophrenia (Holt & Peveler 2005), and only 5 per cent of the general population (Busche & Holt 2004). Risk factors include: family history of diabetes, physical inactivity, poor diet, smoking and the metabolic effects of antipsychotic medication (Gough & Peveler 2004). Typical antipsychotics, in particular the low potency ones such as chlorpromazine, may induce or make existing diabetes worse (Newcomer et al. 2002). The atypical antipsychotics clozapine and olanzapine are associated with new onset or exacerbating type 2 diabetes, not just through their propensity to cause greater weight gain than other newer agents, but because of their effects on glucose regulation (Newcomer et al. 2002). There are also case reports linking risperidone and quetiapine to impaired glucose tolerance, diabetes and ketoacidosis (Taylor et al. 2007).

Recommended action

Blood glucose should be checked at least annually. It may be more practical to do a random test, though a fasting one will be more accurate. The World Health Organisation (2011) recommends that HbAIc can also be used as a diagnostic test for diabetes, providing that stringent quality assurance tests are in place and assays are standardised to criteria aligned to the international reference values, and there are no conditions present that preclude its accurate measurement.

- More frequent assessments are required for people with significant risk factors for diabetes, such as those who are overweight or of Asian/African ethnicity (Barnett *et al.* 2007). Consider checking these patients every six months.
- Offer support and information on diet (e.g. meal planning) and exercise.
- If diabetes is diagnosed or the person has existing diabetes, refer to the practice nurse who specialises in diabetes for the appropriate investigations, education and treatment.

■ ■ ■ Other blood tests to consider

Prolactin

Rationale

Hyperprolactinaemia is a common side effect of many antipsychotic drugs. Symptoms include gynaecomastia, galactorrhoea, amenorrhoea and sexual dysfunction. Switching to a prolactin-sparing antipsychotic has been shown to lead to normalisation of serum prolactin and resolution of the symptoms (Haddad *et al.* 2001).

Recommended action

Consensus guidelines for managing prolactinaemia (Peveler *et al.* 2008) recommend that healthcare professionals should monitor proactively for hyperprolactinaemia, as it may be asymptomatic.

- Patients prescribed prolactin-elevating antipsychotics should, where possible, have this issue explained to them before commencing treatment and be screened for symptoms that suggest hyperprolactinaemia before starting treatment (Haddad *et al.* 2001). The test should be repeated three months later. If there is no change in drug treatment and prolactin levels are within normal range then there is no need to repeat the test.
- If the elevation of prolactin levels is mild (< 1000mIU/L (~ 50ng/mL)), then it may be reasonable to continue to monitor the level. However, if even a mildly elevated level persists for more than three months, particularly if accompanied by amenorrhoea, bone mineral density may be compromised. In this case, the possibility of reducing the dose, or switching to an antipsychotic with lower potential for prolactin elevation, should be discussed with the patient. Consider measuring sex hormones (such as testosterone or oestrogen).
- When elevation is persistent and > 1000mIU/L (~ 50ng/mL) then the clinician should consider switching to a drug with a lower potential to elevate prolactin if this can be achieved safely and is consistent with the patient's overall clinical status.

- For female patients, switching to a drug with a lower potential to elevate prolactin may result in the return of fertility, and contraceptive advice should be given.
- If switching to a drug with a lower potential to elevate prolactin is not possible, it would be reasonable for clinicians to consider offering an oral contraceptive to female patients with amenorrhoea, if this is not contraindicated, to reduce the risk of subsequent osteoporosis.
- In any patient with a prolactin elevation greater than 3000mIU/L (~ 150ng/mL), a prolactinoma should be considered.
- If the levels do not return to normal upon switching to a less prolactin-elevating antipsychotic, or if such as a switch is not possible for clinical reasons, referral to a specialist in endocrinology is warranted to exclude a prolactinoma.

You should also consider other possible causes of hyperprolactinaemia (such as pregnancy or hypothyroidism).

Urea and electrolytes (U&Es) and calcium

Rationale

There is a risk of electrolyte imbalance when taking antipsychotic medication, particularly at high doses. For people taking lithium, there is a higher than normal incidence of hypercalcaemia and abnormal renal function (British National Formulary 2014).

Recommended action

- Check U&Es and calcium annually or when presented with symptoms.
- For people taking lithium, six-monthly checks are recommended (British National Formulary 2014).

Thyroid function test

Rationale

Studies have indicated that the elevated serum levels of T4 may be specific for acutely ill schizophrenic individuals and that neuroleptic medication may affect thyroid hormone metabolism (Baumgartner et al. 2000) and that there is a spectrum of thyroid function test abnormalities in chronic schizophrenia (Othman et al. 1994).

For those taking lithium, there is a higher than normal incidence of hypothyroidism (British National Formulary 2014).

Recommended action

- Check thyroid function annually or in the presence of symptoms.
- For people taking lithium, six-monthly checks are recommended (British National Formulary 2014).

Full blood count (FBC)

Rationale

A case-control study (Teixeira et al. 2009) in people with schizophrenia showed a significantly higher number of people with changes on leukocytes. Many people presented low values of haemoglobin, erythrocytes and platelets. Leukopenia and neutropenia are recognised side effects of antipsychotic medication (Taylor et al. 2007).

Recommended action

Check FBC annually or in the presence of symptoms.

B$_{12}$ and Folate

Rationale

A case-control study (Teixeira et al. 2009) in people with schizophrenia found low values of vitamin B$_{12}$. Having a deficiency of vitamin B$_{12}$ just because of eating a poor diet is rare in Western countries, but unhealthy diets are common in people with schizophrenia (McCreadie 2003).

Recommended action

Check B$_{12}$ and folate annually or in the presence of symptoms.

Vitamin D

Rationale

Most of our vitamin D is made in the skin by the action of sunlight; therefore people who do not go outside are at risk. Vitamin D deficiency is associated with incident cardiovascular disease. Correction of vitamin D deficiency could therefore contribute to the prevention of cardiovascular disease (Wang et al. 2008).

Recommended action

Monitor vitamin D levels every year or if the patient has symptoms (such as tiredness and aching). Advise patients to get exposure to sunlight. Offer supplements if levels are low or the patient is at risk.

Lithium

Rationale

There is potential toxicity caused by lithium therapy when the serum levels are outside the narrow therapeutic range (British National Formulary 2014).

Recommended action

It is recommended that lithium levels are monitored every three months (British National Formulary 2014).

Screening			
Item 9 Prostate and testicular examination (Men only)	*Score*	*Green* Once a month (testicular self-examination)	*Red* Never

Rationale

Cancer of the testicles accounts for only about 1 per cent of all cancers in men. It is, however, the most common type of cancer in males aged 16 to 35, and can occur at any time after the age of 15. Often, only one testicle is affected (Cancer Research 2013a).

Prostate cancer is the most common cancer in men in the UK, with over 40,000 new cases diagnosed every year. It usually develops slowly, so there may be no signs for many years. There is no single test for prostate cancer. It is diagnosed from a blood test, prostate-specific antigen (PSA), a physical examination of the prostate (known as a digital rectal examination or DRE) and a biopsy. Men are not routinely offered PSA tests to screen for prostate cancer, as results can be unreliable.

Recommended action

- Offer information on testicular self-examination (Cancer Research UK 2013a). How to do a testicular self-examination (leaflet): http://www.cancerresearchuk.org/about-cancer/type/testicular-cancer/about/finding-testicular-cancer-early
- If any abnormalities are found, advise the individual to make an appointment with their GP. Advise people in at-risk groups (men aged 50 or older, those of Afro-Caribbean or African descent, and those who have a first degree male relative with prostate cancer) to discuss the benefits of testing for prostate cancer with their GP.

Item 9 Cervical cytology (Women only)	*Score*	*Green* ≤ 3 years (aged 25–64) ≤ 5 years (aged 50–64)	*Red* > 3 years (aged 25–64) > 5 years (aged 50–64)

Rationale

According to the Disability Rights Commission (2006), women with schizophrenia have a lower cervical cancer screening rate (63 per cent) than those without severe mental health problems (73 per cent). However, the evidence shows that if a woman has never been sexually active, her risk of developing cervical cancer is very low indeed (NHS Cancer Screening Programmes 2009a).

Cervical screening saves approximately 4,500 lives per year in England (Peto et al. 2004) and prevents up to 3,900 cases of cervical cancer per year in the UK (Sasieni et al. 1996). Cervical cancer incidence fell by 42 per cent between 1988 and 1997 in England and Wales. This fall is directly related to the cervical screening programme (National Statistics 2000).

Recommended action

- Determine the woman's history of cervical cytology.
- Under 25 years – no screening; 25–49 years – three yearly; 50–64 years – five yearly; 65+ years – those who have not been screened since the age of 50 or have had recent abnormal tests.
- If no recent cervical cytology and the woman has been sexually active, offer an appointment with the practice nurse.

Item 10 Teeth	Score	Green ≤ 12 months	Red ≥ 2 years

Rationale

Antipsychotics, antidepressants and mood stabilisers can cause reduced saliva flow, leading to caries, gingivitis and periodontal disease (Robson & Gray 2007). Dental health may also be affected by poor diet and oral hygiene, and smoking (Friedlander & Marder 2002).

The extent of dental disease can be directly related to schizophrenia intensity, impact of negative symptoms and the length of hospitalisation (Thomas et al. 1996).

Recommended action

- Enquire about oral hygiene and give the appropriate advice.
- Dental check-ups should be every three months to two years, depending on need (DH 2009). People with severe mental illness should be encouraged to make regular visits to the community dentist (NICE 2004a).

Item 11 Eyes	Score	Green ≤ 12 months	Red ≥ 2 years

Rationale

Antipsychotic medication may cause lens and cornea damage, and has been associated with cataract development (Robson & Gray 2007).

Recommended action

People with SMI should be encouraged to visit a local optician/optometrist routinely every two years.

Item 12 Feet	Score	Green Self-check occasionally	Red Never check

Rationale

Some people with SMI struggle to maintain their personal care. Lack of proper care, ill-fitting shoes and general foot neglect are responsible for the majority of foot problems. Feet are the foundation of the body, so if the foot is not functioning correctly, ankles, knees, hips and lower back are not aligned correctly and problems can develop throughout the entire body.

Recommended action

- Offer information on keeping feet healthy, such as washing daily, trimming nails, treatment for burns, cuts and breaks in the skin (Society of Chiropodists and Podiatrists 2005).
- Elderly people or those with diabetes, osteoarthritis and/or rheumatoid arthritis should be a priority in NHS foot care, and should receive regular check-ups from a registered chiropodist (Society of Chiropodists and Podiatrists 2007).
- If the person is presenting any signs/symptoms of foot problems, refer to the chiropodist.

Item 13 Breast examination	Score	Green Women: Self-check monthly/ routine breast screenings Men: Self-check occasionally	Red Never check

Rationale

Breast cancer is the most common cancer in women in the UK (Breast Cancer Care 2010). Hyperprolactinaemia can be an adverse effect of antipsychotic therapy that leads to breast-related problems (Halbreich et al. 2003). The causes of breast cancer in men are not fully known. However, the most important risk factor is increasing age. Most men who get breast cancer are over 60, although younger men can also be affected (Breast Cancer Care 2008).

Recommended action

Everyone should be advised on self-examination (Breast Cancer Care 2010).

- Teach the breast awareness five-point code:
  1. Know what is normal for you.
  2. Know what changes to look and feel for.
  3. Look and feel.
  4. Report any changes to your GP without delay.
  5. Attend routine breast screening if you are a woman aged 50 or over.
- Check risk factors for breast cancer (e.g. previous history, family history, age) (Patient UK 2007).
- If there are any breast abnormalities, refer for further investigations (Patient UK 2007).
- Check for increased levels of serum prolactin (Halbreich et al. 2003).

Item 14 Menstrual cycle (Women only)	Score	Green Regular 28-day ovulation cycle (range: 24–35 days)	Red Irregular/Absent/ Reduced/Excessive

Rationale

Hyperprolactinaemia can cause amenorrhoea, which is associated with anovulation (absence of ovulation) and infertility.

Recommended action

- Check for amenorrhoea – consider offering an oral contraceptive, if this is not contraindicated, to reduce the risk of subsequent osteoporosis. Consider the possibility of pregnancy and test for this if appropriate.
- Check for increased levels of serum prolactin, disturbed menstrual cycle and irregular menstrual cycle (Halbreich et al. 2003). Also see Blood Tests – prolactin (p. XX).

Item 15 Urine	Score	Green 1–2 litres/day	Red < 1litre/day > 3 litres/day

Rationale

Many conditions and chronic urinary tract infections can be detected by using medical urine test strips, and the amount of urine produced can indicate certain conditions.

- Polyuria is the passing of excessive volumes of urine and may be a sign of diabetes, renal failure, alcohol and drug misuse, metabolic abnormalities (Patient UK 2005) and polydipsia.
- Oliguria is reduced urine volume. The cause may be due to dehydration, vascular collapse or low cardiac output (Patient UK 2008).
- Nocturnal enuresis is a less frequently reported side effect of the antipsychotic clozapine (Aronowitz et al. 1995).

Recommended action

- Assess for signs of dehydration (NHS Choices 2013), encourage fluids and implement fluid balance chart to evaluate.
- Assess for symptoms of polyuria (Patient UK 2005) and implement fluid balance chart to evaluate.
- Check for any urine frequency/incontinence issues.
- Dip test urine, using eight parameter (as a minimum) diagnostic strips. Follow the usual protocols for abnormalities.

Item 16 Bowels	Score	Green No constipation/diarrhoea No excessive urgency/ straining/need for laxatives	Red Diarrhoea, constipation, excessive urgency, straining, laxative use

Rationale

A cohort analysis showed that the incidence of colorectal cancer did not differ significantly in people with SMI, compared with the general population (Osborn *et al.* 2013). However, it may be that the cancer is not identified due to the person not presenting with the problem. People with schizophrenia seldom complain of gastrointestinal symptoms unless they are specifically asked (Gupta *et al.* 1997). Some of the preventative behaviours, such as eating a diet low in red or processed meat and high in fibre, fruit and vegetables and being physically active (Cancer Research UK 2013b), are not common in people with SMI.

Recommended action

- Offer information on increasing physical activity, lowering alcohol and a healthy diet.
- The NHS Bowel Cancer Screening Programme offers screening every two years to all men and women aged 60 to 69 (NHS Cancer Screening Programmes 2009b).
- Check for signs of irritable bowel symptoms, diarrhoea or constipation, excessive urgency, gastrointestinal symptoms, straining, bleeding, need for laxatives.
- Check for any bowel frequency/incontinence issues.
- Rapid referral for endoscopy if symptoms are suspicious (NICE 2004b).

Lifestyle			
Item 17 Sleep	Score	Green 7–8 hours	Red < 3 hours > 8 hours

Rationale

Most adults need around 7–8 hours of sleep each night (Benson 2006).

- In untreated schizophrenia, profound insomnia can result from psychotic symptoms (Benson 2006).
- Although antipsychotic treatment can reduce insomnia, the side effects of sedation and residual insomnia can occur (Benson 2006).
- Complaints of poor sleep quality are directly related to negative assessments of quality of life (Benson 2006).
- Improved sleep may lead to improved ability to cope with stress, and increased energy (Hofstetter *et al.* 2005).

Recommended action

- Clarify any personal sleep problems (Hofstetter *et al.* 2005).
- Provide education on good sleep hygiene and the benefits of keeping a sleep diary.
- Consider medication review.

Item 18 Smoking	Score	Green Non-smoker	Red Passive smoker/smoker

Rationale

Smoking rates are high in people with SMI (Osborn *et al.* 2013, Vancampfort *et al.* 2013, Mitchell *et al.* 2011). Neurobiological, psychological, behavioural and social factors make it difficult for people with mental illness to stop smoking (Robson & Gray 2007). Smoking cessation medication and other non-pharmacological support can increase abstinence rates in those with mental health problems to as high as those in the general population (Foulds *et al.* 2006, Campion *et al.* 2008). However, those with mental illness have previously been less likely to receive smoking cessation advice in primary care (Phelan *et al.* 2001).

According to NHS Choices (2009), stopping smoking reduces the risk of :
- Developing illness, disability or death caused by cancer, heart or lung disease
- Gangrene or amputation caused by circulatory problems
- Exposing others to secondhand smoke
- Children in the same household suffering from asthma or glue ear
- Infertility levels, and an unhealthy pregnancy and baby
- Breathing difficulties and decreased general fitness
- Less enjoyment of the taste of food.

Recommended action

- Assess current and past smoking behaviour: 'do you smoke?' or 'are you still smoking?'
- Give information on smoking cessation: 'the best way to stop is with specialist support and medication'. Give advice about the possible health risks associated with smoking. Ask about respiratory symptoms; carry out chest examination if appropriate.
- Give support options, referral to NHS Stop Smoking Services if appropriate (DH 2007a) or the primary care clinic's stop smoking service. Offer medication or nicotine replacement therapies.
- Cigarette smoking lowers the levels of many antipsychotic medications (Vázquez & Beltrán 2007). Therefore, if a person stops or reduces their smoking, a medication review should be undertaken:
  - Blood levels of olanzapine and clozapine should be measured before smoking cessation, followed by 25 per cent dose reduction during the first week of cessation and then further blood levels (Taylor *et al.* 2007).
  - Doses of fluphenazine and benzodiazepine should be reduced by up to 25 per cent in the first week of cessation.
  - Tricyclic antidepressants may need to be reduced by 10–25 per cent in the first week (Taylor *et al.* 2007).

Nicotine replacement is available in a variety of forms and strengths to encourage personal preference and acceptability. Combining patch and faster-acting oral NRT improves efficacy. Side effects include mild local irritation of mouth, throat or nose.

Bupropion is associated with seizures and is contraindicated in bipolar affective disorder and epilepsy. It should not be prescribed with drugs that increase the risk of seizures such as tricyclic antidepressants and some antipsychotics. Bupropion can also alter blood levels of medication such as antipsychotics and antidepressants.

Varenicline has been reported to be more effective and have fewer side effects than bupropion (Cahill et al. 2007). However, reports of exacerbation of depression and suicidal ideation are currently being reviewed (Royal College of Psychiatrists and Royal College of General Practitioners 2010).

Item 19	Score	Green	Red
Exercise		30 minutes a day	None

Rationale
People with SMI are more physically inactive than the general population (Brown et al. 1999, McCreadie 2003). Physical activity can have a positive effect on psychological wellbeing in people with schizophrenia (DH 2004).

Recommended action
Assess the person's level of activity. The recommendation for exercise to be of benefit is 30 minutes, five days a week (DH 2004). Help the person make an exercise plan that fits in with their lifestyle and builds up activity gradually. For some individuals, it may be appropriate to refer to an exercise scheme if there is one in your area.

Item 20	Score	Green	Red
Alcohol intake		2–3 units a day	> 3 units a day

Rationale
Alcohol misuse is one of the most common and clinically significant comorbidities among people with SMI (Brunette et al. 2004). There is considerable evidence to support the positive impact of reducing unsafe alcohol consumption on cardiovascular health (NHS Information Centre 2010).

Many antipsychotics can cause sedation and impair alertness, concentration and coordination. The use of alcohol can further increase any impairment (Rethink 2008).

Recommended action
Offer recommendations on sensible daily alcohol intake (DH 2007b):
- Adult women should not regularly drink > 2–3 units of alcohol a day.
- Adult men should not regularly drink > 3–4 units of alcohol a day.

- Women who regularly drink > 6 units a day (or > 35 units a week) and men who regularly drink > 8 units a day (or > 50 units a week) are at highest risk of alcohol-related harm.

Refer to the local alcohol support service.

Item 22 Diet: literacy 5 a day, fat, salt, carbohydrate intake	Score	Green	Red
		5 fruit/veg a day ≤ 70g (f) ≤ 90g (m) fat a day ≤ 6g salt a day ≤ 230g (f) ≤ 300g (m) carbs a day	≤ 2 fruit/veg a day ≥ 70g (f) ≥ 90g (m) fat a day ≥ 6g salt a day ≥ 230g (f) ≥ 300g (m) carbs a day

Rationale

In a survey of the dietary habits of 102 people with SMI by McCreadie (2003), the average fruit and vegetable intake for these people was 16 portions a week, compared with the recommended intake of 35 per week (DH 2004). The physical health consequences of a poor diet include CVD, diabetes, obesity and some cancers. Studies of people with SMI repeatedly show that saturated fats from dietary intake of meat and dairy products are associated with worse outcomes in schizophrenia (Peet 2004). There is a particularly strong association between sugar consumption and poorer outcome in schizophrenia, whereas consumption of fish and seafood, particularly omega 3 fatty acids, has been associated with better outcomes (Peet 2004).

Recommended action

Agree and implement a diet plan with the person (and any carers). This may include referral to other members of the multidisciplinary team.

- Explain that five portions of fruit/vegetables each day reduces the risk of cancer, coronary heart disease, and other chronic illnesses (DH 2007c).
- Explain that reducing fat intake reduces the risk of cancer, coronary heart disease and other chronic illnesses (DH 2007c).
- Aim to address potential barriers (such as access to and availability of fresh fruit/vegetables, awareness of health benefits and attitudes towards buying, preparing and eating fruit/vegetables) (DH 2007c).

Item 21 Diet: function	Score	Green	Red
		Able to cook and shop Access to cooking facilities	Unable to cook or shop No access to cooking facilities

Rationale

People with SMI may not have access to adequate cooking facilities or have the skills to plan and prepare meals.

Recommended action

Agree and implement a plan with the patient (and carers if appropriate). This may include referral to other members of the multidisciplinary team, such as the occupational therapist for meal planning, shopping and cooking skills.

Item 23 Fluid intake	Score	Green 1–2 litres a day	Red < 1 litre a day > 3 litres a day

Rationale

Many people with severe mental illness do not drink enough fluid and this can lead to dehydration. The body works less efficiently, even with a relatively low level of fluid loss (NHS Choices 2013). Some of the early warning signs are feeling thirsty and light-headed, and having concentrated, strong-smelling urine.

Overconsumption of fluid can also arise from a condition called polydipsia, which is a serious complication of some psychotic illnesses, including schizophrenia. The exact reason for any one person developing polydipsia is unclear, but if untreated, the high intake of fluids can lead to hyponatraemia, which in turn can lead to coma or even death. It has been estimated that between 6 per cent and 17 per cent of psychiatric inpatients suffer from polydipsia (Brooks & Ahmed 2007).

Recommended action

First determine the person's daily fluid intake then follow actions recommended by NHS Choices (2013). If < 1 litre/day:

- Check for signs of dehydration
- Encourage the person to drink 1–2 litres (6–8 glasses) of fluid every day (more during hot weather and physical exertion)
- Offer information on increasing fluid intake (drinking semi-skimmed milk, diluted fruit juices, diluted fruit squash).

If > 3 litres/day:

- Check for signs of polydipsia (Brooks & Ahmed 2007) such as increased urine output
- Implement a fluid balance chart if possible; enlist help of carers and family
- Electrolyte assessment if initial intervention is unsuccessful.

Item 24 Caffeine intake	Score	Green 200–500 mg/day	Red ≥ 600mg/day

Rationale

Caffeine is a central stimulant – in other words, it stimulates the brain. Caffeine is present in drinks such as coffee, tea and cola (NWMHP 2013). Too much caffeine can cause feelings of anxiety and nervousness, sleep disruption (especially difficulty getting off to sleep), restlessness, irritability, increased diuresis, stomach complaints, tremulousness, palpitations and arrhythmias (NWMHP 2013). A moderate daily caffeine intake of 250–500mg is not associated with adverse events (NWMHP 2013). However, psychosis can be induced in normal individuals ingesting caffeine at toxic doses, and psychotic symptoms can also be worsened in patients with schizophrenia who are using caffeine (Broderick & Benjamin 2004).

Table 7.2: Main caffeine-containing foods and drinks

Food or drink item	Average caffeine content
I cup of coffee	75–100mg
I cup of tea	50mg
I can of cola	40mg
I energy drink	90mg
Bar of plain chocolate	50mg
Bar of milk chocolate	25mg

Adapted from Food Standards Agency (2004)

Recommended action
- Offer the person information on reducing caffeine intake and stopping gradually to avoid withdrawal effects (NWMHP 2013).
- Check for symptoms of caffeinism or caffeine toxicity (> 1000mg/day), which can make illnesses such as anxiety more resistant to drug treatment (NWMHP 2013).

Item 25 Cannabis	Score	Green Never	Red Occasional/Regular

Rationale
Cannabis use is associated with poor outcomes in existing schizophrenia (Henquet *et al.* 2005). Cannabis use is a contributing factor in 10 per cent of schizophrenia cases and there are 1,500 expected new cases of cannabis-related schizophrenia each year.

Recommended action
- The individual's cannabis use should be recorded during a physical health check.
- Ask them about other non-prescribed drug use.
- Work with the support of dual diagnosis worker/service – systemically evaluate using a drug use scale.
- Implement health behaviour interventions.

Item 26	Score	Green	Red
Safe sex		Always	Inconsistently/never

Rationale

Although a smaller proportion of people with SMI are sexually active, compared to the general population, those that are sexually active are more likely to engage in high-risk behaviours that may lead to infection with human immunodeficiency virus (HIV), such as sex without a condom and injecting drug use (Cournos et al. 2005). Reasons for this include lack of knowledge about how sexually transmitted diseases (STIs) and HIV are transmitted and prevented (Arrufo et al. 1990, Kalichman et al. 1994), a susceptibility to being coerced into unwanted sexual activity, difficulties in establishing stable social and sexual relationships, and comorbid alcohol and substance use (Coverdale & Turbott 2000).

Recommended action

- Identify whether the person is engaging in behaviours that increase the risk of STIs.
- Provide sexual health advice.
- If STI is suspected, refer to the Genito-Urinary Medicine Clinic.

Item 27	Score	Green	Red
Sexual satisfaction		Satisfied	Dissatisfied

Rationale

Studies show that depression and schizophrenia are associated with impairment of sexual function and satisfaction, whether or not patients are treated with medication (Baldwin & Mayers 2003). That said, antipsychotic medication can have an adverse effect on sexual function, which impacts greatly on quality of life (Hanssens et al. 2006). Smith et al. (2002) showed that sexual dysfunction occurred in 45 per cent of people taking antipsychotic medication; the main cause in both men and women was hyperprolactinaemia. Other medications such as atenolol (for lowering blood pressure), CVD and other physical illness, and a poor relationship with their sexual partner, will also affect sexual function.

Recommended action

- Determine the person's level of sexual activity – refer for gynaecological examination and laboratory assessments if required (EAU 2005).
- Use side effects scale for antipsychotic medication such as the Glasgow Antipsychotic Side-effect Scale (GASS).
- Perform systemic assessment such as the Arizona Sexual Experience Scale – go to: www.psy-world.com/asex_print.htm (McGahuey et al. 2000).
- Check for increased levels of serum prolactin, decreased libido and arousal, orgasmic dysfunction (Halbreich et al. 2003).

■ ■ ■ Medication review

The medication prescribed for people with mental illness has many potential side effects. Carrying out a physical health check also provides the opportunity to perform a medication review.

Antidepressants

The most commonly prescribed antidepressants in primary care are selective serotonin reuptake inhibitors (SSRIs). The most frequent adverse effects associated with these are: nausea, diarrhoea, dizziness, agitation, insomnia, tremor, sweating and sexual dysfunction. The risk of gastrointestinal bleeding is increased in patients taking SSRIs. Other antidepressants, such as venlafaxine can raise blood pressure, and mirtazapine can cause weight gain.

Antipsychotics

Antipsychotics have a wide range of side effects. The most widely researched include: sedation, weight gain, sexual dysfunction and movement disorders (such as dystonia, akathisia, parkinsonian movement disorders, tardive dyskinesia).

Mood stabilisers

In long-term use, lithium has been associated with thyroid disorders and mild cognitive and memory impairment. Lithium salts have a narrow therapeutic/toxic ratio. Therefore it is important to determine the optimum range for each individual patient. Lithium toxicity is made worse by sodium depletion.

In order to be effective, carbamazepine has to reach a certain level in the blood. Side effects include: dizziness, drowsiness, tremor and nausea. Carbamazepine can cause a chronic low white blood cell count, which increases susceptibility to infection. Valproate causes an increase in appetite and can therefore lead to weight gain. Side effects include: dizziness, drowsiness, tremor, nausea, impaired liver function, thrombocytopenia and impaired platelet function.

Recommended action

- Monitor medication use, adherence and side effects (NICE 2013).
- The accuracy of other medication can be checked at the same time as reviewing the antidepressants, antipsychotics and/or mood stabilisers.
- In patients taking an SSRI, check whether they are also being prescribed any drugs that may cause gastrointestinal bleeding (such as triptan, warfarin, heparin, non-steroidal anti-inflammatory drugs, or aspirin). If they are, discuss with GP.
- Blood tests should be taken as described in the blood test section above (see p. 42).
- In patients taking antipsychotics, use a recognised tool such as the Glasgow Antipsychotic Side-effect Scale (GASS). This is a self-rating tool completed by the patient.
- Sedation may be dealt with by the patient taking their medication at night just before they go to bed. The dose may need to be reduced or changed if this is a big problem.

Refer back to the original prescriber in the case of:

- Observed side effects
- Return of symptoms
- Any physical problems that may be related to the prescribed drug
- Any issues flagged up by the patient.

All women with childbearing potential who take psychotropic medication should be encouraged to discuss pregnancy plans with their healthcare professional. They should be made aware of the potential effects of the medications in pregnancy (including the risks of relapse, damage to the foetus, and the risks associated with stopping or changing medication) regardless of whether they are planning a pregnancy. The Scottish Intercollegiate Guidelines Network (SIGN 2013) offers specific guidance for practitioners:

- Discuss the use of reliable contraceptive methods.
- Treat women taking antipsychotics during pregnancy as high risk for gestational diabetes and monitor them for blood glucose abnormalities.
- Advise women who are taking clozapine not to breastfeed.

Changing behaviour to improve health

As discussed in Chapter 6, people with SMI often display a number of unhealthy behaviours. If these are changed, the risk of CVD and other physical conditions will be reduced. You can help people with SMI to change the following unhealthy behaviours:

- Smoking
- Unhealthy eating
- Low levels of physical activity
- Excess consumption of alcohol
- Failure to take medication as prescribed
- Unsafe sex
- Drug misuse.

Before helping someone to change an unhealthy behaviour, you need to assess their readiness to change. The way they react will depend on which stage they are at. The Transtheoretical Model of Change (Prochaska *et al.* 1994) is a model that can be used to assess people's readiness to change any behaviour. There are six stages:

1. *Precontemplation* – They do not intend to make any changes in the near future (usually defined as within the next six months). They are not aware that their behaviour is producing negative consequences. People at this stage may underestimate the benefits of changing their behaviour and think more about the disadvantages of changing it.

2. *Contemplation* – They intend to start the healthy behaviour in the near future. They recognise that their behaviour may be producing negative consequences. They have started to think about the pros and cons of changing the behaviour, giving equal emphasis to each. However, even with this recognition, they may still feel ambivalent about making any changes.

3. *Preparation (Determination)* – They are ready to make changes (within the next 30 days). They start to take small steps towards the behaviour change and believe this can lead to a healthier life.

4. *Action* – They have recently changed their behaviour (within the last six months) and intend to continue with this change. They may show this by modifying their unhealthy behaviour or acquiring new healthy behaviours.

5. *Maintenance* – They have continued their behaviour change (for more than six months) and intend to maintain this change. They work to prevent relapse to earlier stages.

6. *Termination* – They have no desire to return to their unhealthy behaviours and they are sure they will not relapse. This stage is often not considered, as most people tend to stay in the maintenance stage.

■ ■ ■ How to motivate change in people with SMI

Motivational interviewing (MI) is a method of consultation that will help you determine the person's readiness to change and subsequently react in the appropriate manner. It is a directive, client-centred counselling style that aims to help people to explore and resolve ambivalence about behaviour change. It combines elements of style (warmth and empathy) with technique (reflective listening and the development of discrepancy). Ideally, we should use these brief MI techniques to enhance people's motivation to make positive changes via a gentle process of negotiation in which the person is encouraged to discover and articulate for themselves the benefits and costs of change.

There are four central principles of MI:

I. Express empathy by listening and reflecting. Repeat clearly what the person says to you and check that you have understood them correctly. This enables you to convey that you understand not only the person's point of view but also their underlying drivers and motivations.

2. By using open questions and reflection, you can highlight the discrepancies that exist between their most deeply held values and their current behaviour (i.e. tease out ways in which current unhealthy behaviour conflicts with the wish to change). Ask them questions that require more than a 'yes' or 'no' answer – for example, 'What are you hoping to get out of this discussion with me? What do you think about your health?' They may take a while to think about the answer; give them time and don't be afraid of the silence.

3. Avoid conflict by responding with empathy and understanding. Don't say 'You should do this'. This may prevent them coming to see you again in the future.

4. Support self-efficacy by building the person's sense of confidence that change is possible.

By using this approach, you can identify the person's stage of readiness and then consider the most appropriate therapeutic intervention. For example, if the person is really not sure about giving up smoking and is in precontemplation or contemplation, you should acknowledge this by listening, empathising and being curious about their reasons. You should not jump in and provide them with education about nicotine patches until they voice a wish to change. However, if the person is in action, then it will be appropriate to offer them support to help them change their behaviour.

You should try and build their confidence that change is possible but if they don't want to change at this point in time you should not judge them. Simply show that you understand their difficulties, and let them know you are available to help them if they wish to make changes in the future.

Responses that may help you establish the person's readiness to change are described below, along with your role in each situation.

First stage of change – Precontemplation

Person's response: *'I don't want to stop smoking; I'm happy with my weight; I don't feel like changing what I eat.'*

As the person has no interest in changing, there is very little point in giving health information. You should be curious, talk and look for discrepancies, and listen for any clues that they may be willing to change. If any interest is shown, then ask permission to offer advice.

Here's an example:
Person with SMI: *'I can't eat fruit and vegetables because they upset my tummy.'*

Response that might cause conflict: *'You could try introducing fruit and vegetables into your diet slowly.'* If the person is not ready they will respond defensively with lots of reasons why they cannot take on your suggestion. This is where conflict can occur.

Response to avoid conflict: *'Oh dear, that's not nice. Which fruit and vegetables have you tried that affected your stomach?'* and/or *'Does it depend on how much you have?'* Wait for response. *'Are you aware of any fruit and vegetables at all that won't affect your stomach?'*

Second stage of change – Contemplation

Person's response: *'I suppose I would look nicer if I lost weight, but dieting is hard work.'*

Here there is some interest in making a change. The person is able to receive information and to discuss barriers. You should be curious and amplify any discussion of change. Consider working through the pros and cons of making a change and, importantly, the benefits and costs of staying just as they are.

Third stage of change – Preparation and action

Person's response: *'I think I might be fitter if I stopped smoking; what can the doctor give me to help?'*

The person is planning to change and preparing to have a go. You should remain curious, refer to leaflets and evidence, tell stories and use narratives. Help the person to set a target. Planning a target behaviour will give them something specific to aim for. You should do this in partnership with the person. It is helpful to discuss the pros and cons of a possible target behaviour, as this may help them overcome initial resistance. Writing down the pros and cons can make it clearer.

Achievement is more likely if one target is set at a time. You should relate the target to a behaviour (something that the person does), such as walking, rather than an outcome, such as weight loss. The target behaviour should be SMART, meaning Specific (who, what, where, when, how often, with whom, in what context), Measurable (establish criteria), Achievable (realistic, attainable, i.e. start small and build up), Relevant (the person understands the link between their target and their desired outcome) and Timely (realistic, what works for the person).

For example, let's say the desired outcome is to lose weight.

The possible behaviours that the person can choose to lose weight are: to increase their physical activity or to change their diet.

The target behaviour is the level reached of the chosen behaviour before the next review (for instance, in two weeks the person will be walking briskly for 15 minutes, three times a week). When you are helping someone with SMI to plan a target behaviour, you should consider whether the person is capable of doing it, will have the opportunity and will be motivated to carry it out. If any one of these elements is lacking, you should encourage the person to aim for a different target behaviour.

Making a plan helps people to achieve their targets. You should encourage the person with SMI to link their actions to established routines where possible (for instance, taking medication with breakfast) or to make the new actions become routine. This takes less effort so success will be more likely.

There are usually four components to the action plan:

- Where the action is going to take place
- When it is going to happen
- Anyone else involved
- And how long the action will take.

People with SMI may benefit from involving others in helping them achieve their targets – for example, going to a stop smoking group or a ramblers or slimming club; exercising with a friend; or planning shopping/meals with a carer, partner, or flatmate. You should suggest that the person includes who will be involved and how in their plan.

Here's an example.

Target behaviour
Susan will walk briskly for 15 minutes, three times a week, with Mary (her next-door neighbour).

Action plan
Get walking clothes ready on Sunday, Tuesday and Thursday night. Call for Mary on Monday, Wednesday and Friday after breakfast. Walk briskly to the post box (which is about 7 or 8 minutes away) and back again.

Recording the action
It is very important that the person with SMI records what they have done in their action plan so

they have a realistic picture of their progress. It helps to avoid over- or under-estimation of what they have actually done. Also, if they have done well, seeing evidence of their success will increase their motivation. Should there be a problem in achieving their target behaviour, this will be identified.

You should help the person decide how their chosen action can best be measured and encourage them to record this in their plan. Explain to them that writing comments to record progress in detail will help them see what is working and what isn't. Make an appointment with them, to review their progress, on a date that matches the target date for their behaviour target.

Reviewing progress

When the person with SMI returns to see you, greet them with an open question such as 'How did you get on last week?' This will give them the opportunity to explain their progress (or lack of progress) as they see it. Don't say 'Did you manage to...?' If they did not reach the set target, this will make them feel that they have failed. You will be looking to see what they have managed to achieve. Once they have described their progress in their own words, ask to see their plan. This will help you understand what they have actually achieved, compared with their perception of what they have achieved.

- If the person with SMI has achieved their target, praise them for their achievement. Then decide together whether to keep the same goal to ensure that they maintain it, or (if appropriate) set a new target behaviour.
- If the person with SMI has partly achieved their target behaviour, congratulate them on their progress and identify what has been learnt from the experience. You can then help them use this information to change their action in order to make further progress towards achieving the goal.
- If the person with SMI has not achieved their target behaviour, you should praise them for any effort made towards achieving their target (see section below on 'Giving positive feedback'). Again, identify what has been learnt from the experience to help you both plan future actions. Discuss other possible actions that may help them achieve the target behaviour. If other actions cannot be identified, set a new target behaviour.

Giving positive feedback

By giving the person with SMI positive feedback, you will promote their engagement and increase their motivation to continue with their plan.

There are two types of feedback you can give:

- General positive feedback: 'It's nice to see you' or 'You did well this week'.
- Specific positive feedback on target behaviour, which can be divided into three forms:
    1. *Behaviour*: 'You've done all your planned walking this week, well done!'
    2. *Effort*: 'Well done – you're really working hard to get those walks in.'
    3. *Outcome*: 'That's great; you're nearly at your target weight!'

Fourth stage of change – maintenance

Person's response: *'I'm losing weight but it is hard work keeping to this diet.'*

You should listen and reflect on their successes. Then offer them more choice regarding ways to achieve or maintain the change. This may be the time to introduce a new target (such as exercise) to complement their diet. You should reflect their success back to them and encourage positive self-talk.

Fifth stage of change – Maintenance (Relapse prevention)

Person's response: *'I'm really missing my crisps and beer'* or *'I'm getting fed-up'.*

Statements like these could mean that the person with SMI is losing motivation.

Your role is to reassure and offer strategies to maintain the changes. Be curious and ask questions like *'What are your thoughts about why you feel this way?'*

Revisit the pros and cons of the decision, and review the target behaviour.

Dealing with relapse

When a person with SMI has relapsed, your role is to assist them to get back on track. Reassure them that change is rarely runs smoothly, as it is a process rather than an event. You are trying to prevent them feeling that they have failed. You should therefore let them know that relapse is in fact an opportunity to learn about the situations that are likely to lead to relapse and what they can do to avoid them. Developing strategies to manage the risky situations will help them get back on track.

Here is an example. Tom's target behaviour was to ride his bike three times a week for half an hour when he got up. He did this for two weeks but had not managed to do this at all for the last two weeks because he got a puncture. The nurse explained that there are often setbacks and asked him if there was a way he could get his tyre fixed. Tom explained that his brother would probably do it but he hadn't got round to ringing him. The nurse asked Tom how he would like to proceed. If he replied that he would ring his brother and get the puncture repaired then he could continue with the same plan. If this was an issue, the nurse would need to explore an alternative plan with Tom.

■ ■ ■ Summary

People with SMI can change unhealthy behaviour. In order to help them do this, they need to be given support that is appropriate to their stage of readiness to change. For this support to be helpful, the healthcare professional's approach should be positive, encouraging and non-judgemental, and the guidance they offer should be clear and appropriate.

■ ■ ■ Appendix 1

Health Improvement Profile (HIP) – Female

Patient ID _____   Other information _____

Date of birth (age)_____

Ethnic classification _____

Weight _____   Height _____

Date _____

Parameter	Level	Green	Red	Recommended action for red group
BMI		18.50–24.99[1]	< 18.50[1] ≥ 25.00*[1]	☐ BMI < 18.50 – refer for further investigations ☐ BMI ≥ 25.00 – advice and support on diet and exercise, referral to local weight/exercise management programme, consider medication review[2]
Waist circumference		< 80cm†[3]	≥ 80cm†[3]	☐ Advice and support on diet and exercise, referral to local weight/ exercise management programme, consider medication review[2]
Pulse		60–100bpm[4]	< 60 bpm /> 100bpm	☐ ECG should be performed[4]
Blood pressure		<140/90[5]	≥140/90[5]	☐ Advice on weight loss (if over-weight) and increased activity, reduction in alcohol intake, improved diet and smoking cessation[5] ☐ Refer to GP for further investigations[5]
Temperature		36–37.5°C[6]	<36°C[7] >37.5°C[7]	☐ If abnormally high and accompanied by fluctuating BP and/or dystonia, consider neuroleptic malignant syndrome ☐ Report to Responsible Medical Officer, refer for further investigations[6]

Liver function (in last 3 months)		≤ 3 months	> 3 months	☐ Ensure that up-to-date LFTs are conducted ☐ Abnormal – refer for further investigations[8] ☐ Slightly abnormal (> 2 times upper limit of normal) – repeat tests in 6 months' time, check alcohol intake, diabetes control and weight loss[8] ☐ Consider medication review[9]
Lipid levels[a]		TC < 5.1 mmol/L LDL – C < 4.1 mmol/L HDL – C > 1.3mmol/L TG < 2.2 mmol/L[2]	TC ≥ 6.2mmol/L LDL – C ≥ 4.1 mmol/L HDL – C < 1.3 mmol/L or TG ≥ 2.2 mmol/L[2]	☐ Refer to GP for appropriate treatment[2]
Glucose		<6.0mmol/L§**[10] <48mmol/mol (between 48 and 58 if person has diabetes)Ø[11]	≥6.0mmol/L§**[10] ≥ 48mmol/mol (between 48 and 58 if person has diabetes)Ø[11]	☐ Check for symptoms of diabetes[2] ☐ Test for urine ketones if symptoms are present[2] ☐ Refer for further investigations and treatment[2]
Cervical smear		≤ 3 years (aged 25–64) ≤ 5 years (aged 50–64)[12]	> 3 years (aged 25–64)[12] > 5 years (aged 50–64)[12]	☐ Refer to GP or specialist practice nurse[11]
Teeth		≤ 12 months[13]	≥ 2 years[13]	☐ Encourage regular visits to community dentist[13]
Eyes		< 2 years[14]	> 2 years[14]	☐ Prompt to self-refer/refer to optometrist if no eye exam in last 2 years
Feet		Self-check occasionally	Never check	☐ Advice on keeping feet healthy[15] ☐ Elderly patients/those with diabetes – refer to chiropodist[15] ☐ If any presenting signs/symptoms – refer to chiropodist
Breast		Self-check monthly/routine breast screenings	Never check	☐ Advice on self-examination[16] ☐ Patients 50–70 years refer for breast screening (repeat every 3 years)[16] ☐ Breast abnormalities – refer for further investigations[17]

Menstrual cycle		Regular 28-day ovulation cycle (range: 24–35 days)[18]	Irregular/Absent/ Reduced/ Excessive[19]	☐ Refer for further investigations
Urine		1–2 litres/day[20]	< 1 litre/day[20] > 2 litres/day[21]	☐ Assess for signs of dehydration[20] ☐ Assess for symptoms of polyuria[21] ☐ Check for any urine frequency/ incontinence issues ☐ Encourage fluids and implement fluid balance chart to evaluate
Bowels		No constipation/ diarrhoea No excessive urgency/ straining/need for laxatives[22]	Diarrhoea, constipation, excessive urgency, straining, laxative use[22]	☐ Encourage fluids ☐ Check for gastrointestinal symptoms ☐ Check for any bowel urgency/ incontinence issues ☐ Refer for further investigations
Sleep		7–8 hours[23]	< 3 hours[23] > 8 hours[23]	☐ Clarify sleep problem ☐ Provide education on good sleep hygiene and benefits of a sleep diary ☐ Consider medication review ☐ Refer if relapse is suspected (refer to Risk and Relapse Plan and take action accordingly)
Smoking status		Non-smoker	Passive smoker/ smoker	☐ Advise that all smoking is associated with significant health risks[24] ☐ Refer to NHS Stop Smoking Services[24]††
Exercise		30 minutes a day	None	☐ Recommend 30 minutes of activity 5 days a week[25] ☐ Follow up at 3 to 6-monthly intervals[25] ☐ Refer to exercise scheme if required[25]
Alcohol intake		2–3 units/day‡‡[26]	> 3 units/day[26]	☐ Offer recommendations on sensible daily alcohol intake[26] (guide to alcohol units[27])
Diet: literacy 5 a day, fat, salt, carbohydrate intake[a]		5 fruit/veg a day §§[28] ≤ 70g*** fat a day[29] ≤ 6g salt a day[30] ≤ 230g carbs a day[29]	≤ 2 fruit/veg a day[28] ≥ 70g fat a day[29] ≥ 6g salt a day[30] ≥ 230g carbs a day[29]	☐ Offer recommendations on reduction of health risks with healthy eating[28] ☐ Agree and implement a plan with the patient (and carers if appropriate)

Diet: function		Able to cook and shop Access to cooking facilities	Unable to cook or shop No access to cooking facilities	☐ Agree and implement a plan with the patient (and carers if appropriate) ☐ Address potential barriers to accessing and eating fruit/vegetables[28] ☐ May include referral to other members of the MDT, e.g. occupational therapist for meal planning, shopping and cooking skills
Fluid intake		1–2 litres/day[31]	< 1 litre/day[31] > 3 litres/day[32]	☐ < 1 litre/day – check for signs of dehydration[31] ☐ Offer advice on increasing fluid intake[31] ☐ > 3 litres/day – check for signs of polydipsia[32] ☐ Implement a fluid balance chart ☐ Refer for electrolyte assessment if initial intervention unsuccessful
Caffeine intake[a]		200–500mg/day[27]†††	≥ 600mg/day[33]	☐ Check for signs of caffeinism or caffeine toxicity (> 1000 mg/day)[33] ☐ Offer advice to gradually reduce caffeine intake and limit withdrawal effects[33]
Cannabis use		Never	Occasional/Regular	☐ Implement health behaviour interventions and evaluate ☐ Work with support of dual diagnosis worker/service ☐ Systemically evaluate action, e.g. using a Drug Use Scale
Safe sex		Always	Inconsistently/Never	☐ Identify if patient is in high risk group for STIs[34] ☐ Identify if patient is engaging in behaviours that increase risk of STIs[34] ☐ Provide sexual health advice ☐ If STI suspected, refer to GP or sexual health practice nurse[34]
Sexual satisfaction		Satisfied	Dissatisfied	☐ Perform systemic assessment (e.g. Arizona Sexual Experience Scale) of the health parameter ☐ Refer for gynaecological investigations/laboratory assessments[35]

a   Where results fall between red and green ranges, increase frequency of monitoring and review.

*   Overweight = BMI > 23.00 in individuals of South Asian origin.[2]

†   BMI for Europids – refer to ethnic-specific values where required.

§**   Fasting plasma glucose.

Ø   glycated haemoglobin.

††   Warning – careful planning/medication review is required if smoking cessation is planned. Mental health nurse to identify this need.

‡‡   Pregnant women should avoid drinking alcohol. If they do choose to drink, they should not drink more than 1–2 units once or twice a week.

§§   Five portions of a variety of fruit and vegetables.

***   A portion of food that is high in saturated fat or trans fat (e.g. meat products, hard cheese, butter/lard, pastry, cakes/biscuits, cream). Total fat content is considered high if the food contains more than 20g fat per 100g.

†††   Average caffeine content – 1 cup of coffee = 75–100mg; 1 cup of tea = 50mg; 1 can of cola = 40mg; 1 energy drink = 90mg; bar of plain chocolate = 50mg; bar of milk chocolate = 25mg.

BMI – body mass index; ECG – electrocardiogram; HDL-C – high density lipoprotein – cholesterol; LDL-C – low density lipoprotein – cholesterol; STI – sexually transmitted infection; TC – total cholesterol; TG – triglycerides; ULN – upper limit of normal.

Other blood tests to consider: prolactin, urea and electrolytes and calcium, thyroid function test, full blood count, B_{12} and folate, lithium levels, Vitamin D.

References to Appendix 1

1. WHO (World Health Organization) (2007). BMI Classification. http://www.who.int/bmi/index.jsp?introPage=intro_3.html (Accessed 30 December 2014).

2. Barnett, A., Mackin, P., Chaudhry, I. et al. (2007). Minimizing metabolic and cardiovascular risk in schizophrenia: diabetes, obesity and dyslipidaemia. *Journal of Psychopharmacology.* **21**, 357–73.

3. International Diabetes Federation (IDF). (2006). The IDF consensus worldwide definition of the metabolic syndrome.

4. British Heart Foundation (BHF). (2007). Abnormal heart rhythms. https://www.bhf.org.uk/heart-health/conditions/abnormal-heart-rhythms (Accessed 30 December 2014).

5. NICE (National Institute for Health and Clinical Excellence) (2011). *CG127 Hypertension: Clinical management of primary hypertension in adults* http://publications.nice.org.uk/hypertension-cg127 (Accessed 30 December 2014).

6. Medline Plus. (Oct 2006). Medical Encyclopaedia: Temperature measurement. http://www.nlm.nih.gov/medlineplus/encyarticle/003400.htm#top (Accessed 30 December 2014).

7. Dougherty, L. & Lister, S. (eds) (2004). *The Royal Marsden Hospital Manual of Clinical Nursing Procedures.* 6th edn. Oxford: Blackwell Publishing.

8. Patient UK (Sep 2006). Abnormal liver function tests. EMIS. http://www.patient.co.uk/doctor/abnormal-liver-function-tests (Accessed 30 December 2014).

9. Garcia-Unzueta, M.T., Herran, A., Sierra-Biddle, D. et al. (2003). Alterations of liver function test in patients treated with antipsychotics. *Journal of Clinical Laboratory Analysis.* **17**, 216–18.

10. WHO (World Health Organization) (2011). Use of Glycated Haemoglobin (HbAlc) in the Diagnosis of Diabetes Mellitus. http://www.diabetes.org.uk/Documents/Professionals/hba1c_diagnosis.1111.pdf (Accessed 30 December 2014).

11. NICE (National Institute for Health and Clinical Excellence) (2011). PH35 Preventing type 2 diabetes: population and community-level interventions in high-risk groups and the general population. http://www.nice.org.uk/guidance/PH35/Guidance/pdf (Accessed 30 December 2014).

12. Patient UK (May 2007). Cervical screening test. EMIS. http://www.patient.co.uk/showdoc/23068699/ (Accessed 30 December 2014).

13. NICE (National Institute for Health and Clinical Excellence). (Oct 2004). CG19 Dental Recall. Recall interval between routine dental examinations.

14. NHS Choices (2012). Why are regular eye tests (sight tests) so important? http://www.nhs.uk/Livewell/Eyehealth/Pages/Lookingafteryoureyes.aspx (Accessed 30 December 2014).

15. NHS Choices (2013). Foot problems and the podiatrist. http://www.nhs.uk/Livewell/foothealth/Pages/Foot-problems-podiatrist.aspx (Accessed 30 December 2014).

16. Breast Cancer Care (May 2000). Breast awareness. http://www.breastcancercare.org.uk (Accessed 30 December 2014).

17. Patient UK (Apr 2007). Breast lumps and breast examination. EMIS. http://www.patient.co.uk/showdoc/40000260/ (Accessed 30 December 2014).

18. NHS Choices (2014). Periods and fertility in the menstrual cycle. http://www.nhs.uk/Livewell/menstrualcycle/Pages/Whatisthemenstrualcycle.aspx (Accessed 30 December 2014).

19. GPnotebook. Abnormal menstrual bleeding. http://www.gpnotebook.co.uk/simplepage.cfm?ID=1033502758 (Accessed 30 December 2014).

20. NHS Choices (2013). Dehydration. http://www.nhs.uk/conditions/dehydration/pages/introduction.aspx (Accessed 30 December 2014).

21. Patient UK (2005). Polyuria. EMIS. http://www.patient.co.uk/showdoc/40000113 (Accessed 30 December 2014)

22. Cancer Research UK (Jan 2007). About the bowel. http://www.cancerhelp.org.uk/help/default.asp?page=14326 (Accessed 30 December 2014).

23. The Sleep Council (2012). Sleep advice. http://www.sleepcouncil.org.uk/how-to-sleep/ (Accessed 30 December 2014).

24. Department of Health (2008). NHS Stop Smoking Services & Nicotine Replacement Therapy. http://webarchive.nationalarchives.gov.uk/+/www.dh.gov.uk/en/Publichealth/Healthimprovement/Tobacco/Tobaccogeneralinformation/DH_4002192 (Accessed 30 December 2014).

25. NICE (National Institute for Clinical Excellence) (Mar 2006). Public Health Intervention Guidance No. 2. Four commonly used methods to increase physical activity: brief interventions in primary care, exercise referral schemes, pedometers and community-based exercise programmes for walking and cycling. http://www.nice.org.uk/guidance/ph2 (Accessed 30 December 2014).

26. Department of Health. (Jun 2007). *Safe. Sensible. Social. The next steps in the National Alcohol Strategy.* http://webarchive.nationalarchives.gov.uk/20130107105354/http:/www.dh.gov.uk/en/Publicationsandstatistics/Publications/PublicationsPolicyAndGuidance/DH_075218 (Accessed 30 December 2014).

27. Drinkaware (2012). What is an alcohol unit? https://www.drinkaware.co.uk/check-the-facts/what-is-alcohol/what-is-an-alcohol-unit (Accessed 30 December 2014).

28. Department of Health. (Feb 2007). *5 a day introduction.* http://webarchive.nationalarchives.gov.uk/20061016092221/http://dh.gov.uk/en/Policyandguidance/Healthandsocialcaretopics/FiveADay/FiveADaygeneralinformation/index.htm (Accessed 30 December 2014).

29. NHS Choices. (2014). *Salt: the facts.* http://www.nhs.uk/Livewell/Goodfood/Pages/salt.aspx (Accessed 30 December 2014).

30. Food and Drink Federation (2014). *Guideline Daily Amounts.* http://www.gdalabel.org.uk/gda/gda_values.aspx (Accessed 30 December 2014).

31. NHS Choices. Water and drinks http://www.nhs.uk/Livewell/Goodfood/Pages/water-drinks.aspx (Accessed 30 December 2014).

32. Brooks, G. & Ahmed, A.G. (2007). Pharmacological treatment for psychosis related polydipsia (review). *The Cochrane Library.* 3, 1–15.

33. Norfolk and Waveney Mental Health Partnership NHS Trust (NWMHP). NWMHP Pharmacy Medicine Information: caffeine. http://webarchive.nationalarchives.gov.uk/20090305155609/http://www.nwmhp.nhs.uk/pharmacy/caffeine.htm (Accessed 30 December 2014).

34. NICE (National Institute for Health and Clinical Excellence) (Feb 2007). NICE Public Health Intervention Guidance No. 3. One to one interventions to reduce the transmission of sexually transmitted infections (STIs) including HIV, and to reduce the rate of under 18 conceptions, especially among vulnerable and at risk groups. http://www.kernowps.co.uk/guide.pdf (Accessed 30 December 2014).

35. Philip, N.A. (2000). Female sexual dysfunction: evaluation and treatment. *American Family Physician.* 62.

■■■Appendix 2

Health Improvement Profile (HIP) – Male

Patient ID _____   Other information _____

Date of birth (age)_____

Ethnic classification _____

Weight _____   Height _____

Date _____

Parameter	Level	Green	Red	Recommended action for red group
BMI		18.50–24.99[1]	< 18.50[1] ≥ 25.00[1]*	☐ BMI < 18.50 – refer for further investigations ☐ BMI ≥ 25.00 – advice and support on diet and exercise, referral to local weight/exercise management programme, consider medication review[2]
Waist circumference		< 94cm†[3]	≥ 94cm†[3]	☐ Advice and support on diet and exercise, referral to local weight/ exercise management programme, consider medication review[2]
Pulse		60–100bpm[4]	< 60 bpm /> 100bpm	☐ ECG should be performed[4]
Blood pressure		<140/90[5]	≥140/90[5]	☐ Advice on weight loss (if over-weight) and increased activity, reduction in alcohol intake, improved diet and smoking cessation[5] ☐ Refer to GP for further investigations[5]
Temperature		36–37.5°C[6]	<36°C[7] >37.5°C[7]	☐ If abnormally high and accompanied by fluctuating BP and/or dystonia, consider neuroleptic malignant syndrome ☐ Report to Responsible Medical Officer, refer for further investigations[6]

Liver function (in last 3 months)		≤ 3 months	> 3 months	☐ Ensure that up-to-date LFTs are conducted ☐ Abnormal – refer for further investigations[8] ☐ Slightly abnormal (> 2 times upper limit of normal) – repeat tests in 6 months' time, check alcohol intake, diabetes control and weight loss[8] ☐ Consider medication review[9]
Lipid levels		TC < 5.1 mmol/L LDL – C < 4.1 mmol/L HDL – C > 1.0mmol/L TG< 2.2mmol/L[2]	TC ≥ 6.2mmol/L LDL– C ≥ 4.1 mmol/L HDL – C< 1.0mmol/L or TG ≥ 2.2mmol/L[2]	☐ Refer to GP for appropriate treatment[2]
Glucose		<6.0mmol/L§**[10] <48mmol/mol (between 48 and 58 if person has diabetes)Ø[11]	≥ 6.0mmol/L§**[10] ≥ 48mmol/mol (between 48 and 58 if person has diabetes)[11]	☐ Check for symptoms of diabetes[2] ☐ Test for urine ketones if symptoms are present[2] ☐ Refer for further investigations and treatment[2]
Prostate and testicles		Once a month (testicular self-examination)[12]	Never	☐ Confirm prostate screening at fixed intervals for patients over 50 years[13] ☐ No recent PSA test – refer to GP or specialised practice nurse
Teeth		≤ 12 months[14]	≥ 2 years[14]	☐ Encourage regular visits to community dentist[14]
Eyes		< 2 years[15]	> 2 years[15]	☐ Prompt to self-refer/refer to opto-metrist if no eye exam in last 2 years
Feet		Self-check occasionally	Never check	☐ Advice on keeping feet healthy[16] ☐ Elderly patients/those with diabetes – refer to chiropodist[16] ☐ If any presenting signs/symptoms – refer to chiropodist
Breast		Self-check occasionally	Never check	☐ Check risk factors for male breast cancer (i.e. previous radiotherapy, obesity, family history of breast cancer, high oestrogen levels or chromosomal syndromes)[17]

Breast (cont.)			☐ Breast abnormalities – refer for further investigations[17]
Urine	1–2 litres/day[18]	< 1 litre/day[18] > 2 litres/day[19]	☐ Assess for signs of dehydration[18] ☐ Assess for symptoms of polyuria[19] ☐ Check for any urine frequency/ incontinence issues ☐ Encourage fluids and implement fluid balance chart to evaluate
Bowels	No constipation/ diarrhoea No excessive urgency/ straining/need for laxatives[20]	Diarrhoea, constipation, excessive urgency, straining, laxative use[20]	☐ Encourage fluids ☐ Check for gastrointestinal symptoms ☐ Check for any bowel urgency/ incontinence issues ☐ Refer for further investigations
Sleep	7–8 hours[21]	< 3 hours[21] > 8 hours[21]	☐ Clarify sleep problem ☐ Provide education on good sleep hygiene and benefits of a sleep diary ☐ Consider medication review ☐ Refer if relapse is suspected (refer to Risk and Relapse Plan and take action accordingly)
Smoking status	Non-smoker	Passive smoker/ smoker	☐ Advise that all smoking is associated with significant health risks[22] ☐ Refer to NHS Stop Smoking Services[18]††
Exercise	30 minutes a day[23]	None	☐ Recommend 30 minutes of activity 5 days a week[23] ☐ Follow up at 3 to 6-monthly intervals[23] ☐ Refer to exercise scheme if required[23]
Alcohol intake	3–4 units/day[24]	>4 units/day[24]	☐ Offer recommendations on sensible daily alcohol intake[24] (guide to alcohol units[25])
Diet: literacy 5 a day, fat, salt, carbohydrate intake[a]	5 fruit/veg a day §§[26] ≤ 70g*** fat a day[27] ≤6g salt a day[28] ≤230g carbs a day[27]	≤ 2 fruit/veg a day[26] ≥ 70g fat a day[27] ≥6g salt a day[28] ≥230g carbs a day[27]	☐ Offer recommendations on reduction of health risks with healthy eating[26] ☐ Agree and implement a plan with the patient (and carers if appropriate)

Diet: function		Able to cook and shop Access to cooking facilities	Unable to cook or shop No access to cooking facilities	☐ Agree and implement a plan with the patient (and carers if appropriate) ☐ Address potential barriers to accessing and eating fruit/vegetables[26] ☐ May include referral to other members of the MDT, e.g. occupational therapist for meal planning, shopping and cooking skills
Fluid intake		1–2 litres/day[29]	< 1 litre/day[29] > 3 litres/day[30]	☐ < 1 litre/day – check for signs of dehydration[29] ☐ Offer advice on increasing fluid intake[29] ☐ > 3 litres/day – check for signs of polydipsia[30] ☐ Implement a fluid balance chart ☐ Refer for electrolyte assessment if initial intervention unsuccessful
Caffeine intake[a]		200–500mg/day[31]††††	≥ 600mg/day[31]	☐ Check for signs of caffeinism or caffeine toxicity (> 1000 mg/day)[31] ☐ Offer advice to gradually reduce caffeine intake and limit withdrawal effects[31]
Cannabis use		Never	Occasional/Regular	☐ Implement health behaviour interventions and evaluate ☐ Work with support of dual diagnosis worker/service ☐ Systemically evaluate action, e.g. using a Drug Use Scale
Safe sex		Always	Inconsistently/Never	☐ Identify if patient is in high risk group for STIs[32] ☐ Identify if patient is engaging in behaviours that increase risk of STIs[32] ☐ Provide sexual health advice ☐ If STI suspected, refer to GP or sexual health practice nurse[32]
Sexual satisfaction		Satisfied	Dissatisfied	☐ Determine patient's level of sexual activity[33] ☐ Perform systemic assessment (e.g. Arizona Sexual Experience Scale) of the health parameter

a Where results fall between red and green ranges, increase frequency of monitoring and review.

* Overweight = BMI > 23.00 in individuals of South Asian origin.[2]

† BMI for Europids – refer to ethnic-specific values where required.

§** Fasting plasma glucose.

Ø glycated haemoglobin.

†† Warning – careful planning/medication review is required if smoking cessation is planned. Mental health nurse to identify this need.

§§ Five portions of a variety of fruit and vegetables.

*** A portion of food that is high in saturated fat or trans fat (e.g. meat products, hard cheese, butter/lard, pastry, cakes/biscuits, cream). Total fat content is considered high if the food contains more than 20g fat per 100g.

††† Average caffeine content – 1 cup of coffee = 75–100mg; 1 cup of tea = 50mg; 1 can of cola = 40mg; 1 energy drink = 90mg; bar of plain chocolate = 50mg; bar of milk chocolate = 25mg.

BMI – body mass index; ECG – electrocardiogram; HDL-C – high density lipoprotein – cholesterol; LDL-C – low density lipoprotein – cholesterol; STI – sexually transmitted infection; TC – total cholesterol; TG triglycerides; ULN – upper limit of normal.

Other blood tests to consider: prolactin, urea and electrolytes and calcium, thyroid function test, full blood count, B_{12} and folate, lithium levels, Vitamin D.

References to Appendix 2

1. WHO (World Health Organization) (2007). BMI Classification.
http://www.who.int/bmi/index.jsp?introPage=intro_3.html (Accessed 30 December 2014).

2. Barnett, A., Mackin, P., Chaudhry, I. et al. (2007). Minimizing metabolic and cardiovascular risk in schizophrenia: diabetes, obesity and dyslipidaemia. Journal of Psychopharmacology. **21**, 357–73.

3. International Diabetes Federation (IDF). (2006). The IDF consensus worldwide definition of the metabolic syndrome.

4. British Heart Foundation (BHF). (2007). Abnormal heart rhythms.
https://www.bhf.org.uk/heart-health/conditions/abnormal-heart-rhythms (Accessed 30 December 2014).

5. NICE (National Institute for Health and Clinical Excellence) (2011). CG127 Hypertension: Clinical management of primary hypertension in adults http://publications.nice.org.uk/hypertension-cg127

6. Medline Plus. (Oct 2006). Medical Encyclopaedia: Temperature measurement.
http://www.nlm.nih.gov/medlineplus/ency/article/003400.htm#top

7. Dougherty, L. & Lister, S. (eds) (2004). The Royal Marsden Hospital Manual of Clinical Nursing Procedures. 6th edn. Oxford: Blackwell Publishing.

8. Patient UK (Sep 2006). Abnormal liver function tests. EMIS.
http://www.patient.co.uk/doctor/abnormal-liver-function-tests (Accessed 30 December 2014).

9. Garcia-Unzueta, M.T., Herran, A., Sierra-Biddle, D. et al. (2003). Alterations of liver function test in patients treated with antipsychotics. Journal of Clinical Laboratory Analysis. **17**, 216–8.

10. WHO (World Health Organization) (2011). Use of Glycated Haemoglobin (HbA1c) in the Diagnosis of Diabetes Mellitus. http://www.diabetes.org.uk/Documents/Professionals/hba1c_diagnosis.1111.pdf

11. NICE (National Institute for Health and Clinical Excellence) (2011). PH35 Preventing type 2 diabetes: population and community-level interventions in high-risk groups and the general population. http://www.nice.org.uk/guidance/PH35/Guidance/pdf

12. Mistry, R. (2005). Tips on – testicular self examination. *Student British Medical Journal.* **13**, 441–84.
http://student.bmj.com/student/view-article.html?id=sbmj0512462a

13. Prostate Cancer UK. http://prostatecanceruk.org/prostate-information/getting-diagnosed (Accessed 30 December 2014).

14. NICE (National Institute for Health and Clinical Excellence). (Oct 2004). CG19 Dental Recall. Recall interval between routine dental examinations.

15. NHS Choices (2012). Why are regular eye tests (sight tests) so important?
http://www.nhs.uk/Livewell/Eyehealth/Pages/Lookingafteryoureyes.aspx (Accessed 30 December 2014).

16. NHS Choices (2013). Foot problems and the podiatrist.
http://www.nhs.uk/Livewell/foothealth/Pages/Foot-problems-podiatrist.aspx (Accessed 30 December 2014).

17. Breast Cancer Care (2014). Breast cancer in men.
http://www.breastcancercare.org.uk/breast-cancer-information/about-breast-cancer/men-breast-cancer (Accessed 30 December 2014).

18. NHS Choices (2013). Dehydration.
http://www.nhs.uk/conditions/dehydration/pages/introduction.aspx (Accessed 30 December 2014).

19. Patient UK (2005). Polyuria. EMIS. http://www.patient.co.uk/showdoc/40000113/ (Accessed 30 December 2014).

20. Cancer Research UK (Jan 2007). About the bowel.
http://www.cancerhelp.org.uk/help/default.asp?page=14326 (Accessed 30 December 2014).

21. The Sleep Council (2012). Sleep advice. http://www.sleepcouncil.org.uk/how-to-sleep/ (Accessed 30 December 2014).

22. Department of Health (2008). NHS Stop Smoking Services & Nicotine Replacement Therapy.
http://webarchive.nationalarchives.gov.uk/+/www.dh.gov.uk/en/Publichealth/Healthimprovement/Tobacco/Tobaccogeneralinformation/DH_4002192 (Accessed 30 December 2014).

23. NICE (National Institute for Health and Clinical Excellence) (Mar 2006). Public Health Intervention Guidance No. 2. Four commonly used methods to increase physical activity: brief interventions in primary care, exercise referral schemes, pedometers and community-based exercise programmes for walking and cycling.
http://www.nice.org.uk/guidance/ph2 (Accessed 30 December 2014).

24. Department of Health (Jun 2007). *Safe. Sensible. Social. The next steps in the National Alcohol Strategy.*
http://webarchive.nationalarchives.gov.uk/20130107105354/http:/www.dh.gov.uk/en/Publicationsandstatistics/Publications/PublicationsPolicyAndGuidance/DH_075218 (Accessed 30 December 2014).

25. Drinkaware (2012). What is an alcohol unit?
https://www.drinkaware.co.uk/check-the-facts/what-is-alcohol/what-is-an-alcohol-unit (Accessed 30 December 2014).

26. Department of Health. (Feb 2007). *5 a day introduction.*
http://webarchive.nationalarchives.gov.uk/20061016092221/http://dh.gov.uk/en/Policyandguidance/Healthandsocialcaretopics/FiveADay/FiveADaygeneralinformation/index.htm (Accessed 30 December 2014).

27. NHS Choices. (2014). *Salt: the facts.* http://www.nhs.uk/Livewell/Goodfood/Pages/salt.aspx (Accessed 30 December 2014).

28. Food and Drink Federation (2014). *Guideline Daily Amounts.*
http://www.gdalabel.org.uk/gda/gda_values.aspx (Accessed 30 December 2014).

29. NHS Choices. *Water and drinks* http://www.nhs.uk/Livewell/Goodfood/Pages/water-drinks.aspx (Accessed 30 December 2014).

30. Brooks, G. & Ahmed, A.G. (2007). Pharmacological treatment for psychosis related polydipsia (review). *The Cochrane Library.* **3**, 1–15.

31. Norfolk and Waveney Mental Health Partnership NHS Trust (NWMHP). NWMHP Pharmacy Medicine Information: caffeine.
http://webarchive.nationalarchives.gov.uk/20090305155609/http://www.nwmhp.nhs.uk/pharmacy/caffeine.htm (Accessed 30 December 2014).

32. NICE (National Institute for Health and Clinical Excellence) (Feb 2007). NICE Public Health Intervention Guidance No. 3. One to one interventions to reduce the transmission of sexually transmitted infections (STIs) including HIV, and to reduce the rate of under 18 conceptions, especially among vulnerable and at risk groups.
http://www.kernowps.co.uk/guide.pdf (Accessed 30 December 2014).

33. European Association of Urology (EAU) (Mar 2005). *Guidelines on erectile dysfunction.* EAU.

■■■ References

Abdelmawla, M. & Mitchell, A. (2006). Sudden cardiac death and antipsychotics. *Advances in Psychiatric Treatment*. **12**, 100–109.

Abraham, G., Paing, W., Kaminski, J., Joseph, A., Kohegyi, E. & Josiassen, R. (2003). Effects of elevated serum prolactin on bone mineral density and bone metabolism in female patients with schizophrenia: a prospective study. *American Journal of Psychiatry*. **160**, 1618–620.

Aizenberg, D., Zemishlany, Z., Dorfman-Etrog, P. & Weizman, A. (1995). Sexual dysfunction in male schizophrenic patients. *Journal of Clinical Psychiatry*. **56**, 137–41.

Allebeck, P., Adamsson, C. & Engström, A. (1993). Cannabis and schizophrenia: a longitudinal study of cases treated in Stockholm County. *Acta Psychiatrica Scandinavica*. **88**, 21–24.

Allison, D. & Casey, D. (2001). Antipsychotic-induced weight gain. A review of the literature. *Journal of Clinical Psychiatry*. **62** (suppl. 7), 22–31.

American Psychiatric Association (APA) (2013). *The Diagnostic and Statistical Manual of Mental Disorders*. 5th edition. Arlington (VA): APA.

Andreasen, N. (1995). Symptoms, signs and diagnosis of schizophrenia. *The Lancet*. **346** (8973), 453–516.

Aronowitz, J., Safferman, A. & Lieberman, J. (1995). Management of clozapine-induced enuresis. *American Journal of Psychiatry*. **152**, 472–73.

Arrufo, J., Coverdale, J., Chako, R., et al. (1990). Knowledge about AIDS among women psychiatric outpatients. *Hospital and Community Psychiatry*. **41**, 326–28.

Ataya, K., Mercado, A., Kartaginer, J., Abbasi, A. & Moghissi, K. (1988). Bone density and reproductive hormones in patients with neuroleptic-induced hyperprolactinemia. *Fertility and Sterility*. **50**, 876–81.

Atkin, K., Kendall, F., Gould, D., Freeman, H., Liberman, J. & O'Sullivan, D. (1996). Neutropenia and agranulocytosis in patients receiving clozapine in the UK and Ireland. *The British Journal of Psychiatry*. **169**, 483–88.

Baastrup, P., Christiansen, C. & Transbol, I. (1980). Calcium metabolism in schizophrenic patients on long-term neuroleptic therapy. *Neuropsychobiology*. **6**, 56–59.

Bairey Merz, C., Dwyer, J., Nordstrom, C., Walton, K., Salerno, J. & Schneider, R. (2002). Psychosocial stress and cardiovascular disease: Pathophysiological links. *Behavioral Medicine*. **27**, 141–46.

Baldwin, D. & Mayers, A. (2003). Sexual side-effects of antidepressant and antipsychotic drugs. *Advances in Psychiatric Treatment*. **9**, 202–10.

Baldwin, J. (1979). Schizophrenia and physical disease. *Psychological Medicine*. **9** (4), 611–18.

Barak, Y., Achiron, A., Mandel, M., Mirecki, I. & Aizenberg, D. (2005). Reduced cancer incidence among patients with schizophrenia. *Cancer*. **104**, 2817–21.

Barnett, A., Mackin, P., Chaudhry, I., Farooqi, A., Gadsby, R., Heald, A., Hill, J., Millar, H., Peveler, R., Rees, A., Singh, V., Taylor, D., Vora, J. & Jones, P.B. (2007). Minimising metabolic and cardiovascular risk in schizophrenia: diabetes, obesity and dyslipidaemia. *Journal of Psychopharmacology*. **21** (4), 357–73.

Batki, S., Meszaros, Z., Strutynski, K. et al. (2009). Medical comorbidity in patients with schizophrenia and alcohol dependence. *Schizophrenia Research*. **107**, 139–46.

Baumgartnera, A., Pietzckerb, A. & Gaebelc, W. (2000). The hypothalamic–pituitary–thyroid axis in patients with schizophrenia. *Schizophrenia Research*. **44** (3), 233–43.

Bennedsen, B. (1998). Adverse pregnancy outcome in schizophrenic women: occurrence and risk factors. *Schizophrenia Research*. **33**, 1–26.

Benson, K. (2006). Sleep in schizophrenia: impairments, correlates, and treatment. *Psychiatric Clinics of North America*. **29**, 1033–45.

Bergemann, N., Auler, B., Parzer, P. et al. (2001). High bone turnover but normal bone mineral density in women with schizophrenia. *Bone*. **28**, 248.

Bilici, M., Cakirbay, H., Guler, M., Tosun, M., Ulgen, M. & Tan, U. (2002). Classical and atypical neuroleptics, and bone mineral density, in patients with schizophrenia. *International Journal of Neuroscience.* **112**, 817–28.

Bishop, J., Alexander, B., Lund, B. & Klepser, T. (2004). Osteoporosis screening and treatment in women with schizophrenia: a controlled study. *Pharmacotherapy.* **24**, 515–21.

BMA and NHS Employers (2014). QOF Guidance 2014–2015 (seventh revision). http://bma.org.uk/practical-support-at-work/contracts/independent-contractors/qof-guidance (Accessed 30 December 2014).

Breast Cancer Care (2008). Men with breast cancer. http://www.breastcancercare.org.uk/upload/pdf/men_with_breast_cancer_08_web_0.pdf (Accessed 17 December 2014).

Breast Cancer Care (2010). Breast awareness. http://www.breastcancercare.org.uk/breast-cancer-breast-health/breast-awareness/ (Accessed 17 December 2014).

British National Formulary (2014). *BNF 68.* London: Pharmaceutical Press.

Broderick, P. & Benjamin, A. (2004). Caffeine and psychiatric symptoms: A Review. *Journal of Oklahoma State Medical Association.* **97** (12), 538–42.

Brooks, G. & Ahmed, A. (2007). Pharmacological treatments for psychosis-related polydipsia. *The Cochrane Library.* **3**, 1–15.

Brown, S., Birtwistle, J., Roe, L. & Thompson, C. (1999). The unhealthy lifestyle of people with schizophrenia. *Psychological Medicine.* **29**, 697–701.

Brunette, M.F., Mueser, K.T. & Drake, R.E. (2004). A review of research on residential programs for people with severe mental illness and co-occurring substance use disorders. *Drug and Alcohol Review.* **23**, 471–81.

Buhagiar, K., Parsonage, L. & Osborn D. (2011). Physical health behaviours and health locus of control in people with schizophrenia-spectrum disorder and bipolar disorder: a cross-sectional comparative study with people with non-psychotic mental illness. *BMC Psychiatry.* **11**, 104.

Burns, M. (2001). The pharmacology and toxicology of atypical antipsychotic agents. *Journal of Clinical Toxicology.* **39** (1), 1–14.

Busche, B. & Holt, R. (2004). Prevalence of diabetes and impaired glucose tolerance in patients with schizophrenia. *British Journal of Psychiatry.* **184**, S67–S71.

Cahill, K., Stead, L. & Lancaster, T. (2007). Nicotine receptor partial agonists for smoking cessation. *Cochrane Database of Systematic Reviews.* Issue 1, CD006103. Wiley Interscience.

Calabrese, J., Keck, P. Jr, Macfadden, W., Minkwitz, M., Ketter, T., Weisler, R., Cutler, A., McCoy, R., Wilson, E. & Mullen, J. (2005). A randomized, double-blind, placebo-controlled trial of quetiapine in the treatment of bipolar I or II depression. *American Journal of Psychiatry.* **162** (7), 1351–60.

Campion, J., Checinski, K. & Nurse, J. (2008). Review of smoking cessation treatments for people with mental illness. *Advances in Psychiatric Treatment.* **14**, 208–16.

Cancer Research UK. (2013a) Testicular Cancer: key facts. http://www.cancerresearchuk.org/cancer-info/cancerstats/keyfacts/testicular-cancer/ (Accessed 17 December 2014).

Cancer Research UK (2013b). Bowel Cancer: key facts. http://www.cancerresearchuk.org/cancer-info/cancerstats/keyfacts/bowel-cancer/ (Accessed 17 December 2014).

Cardno, A. & Gottesman, I. (2000). Twin studies of schizophrenia: from bow-and-arrow concordances to star wars Mx and functional genomics. *American Journal of Medical Genetics.* **97** (1), 12–17.

Carey, M.P., Carey, K.B., Maisto, S.A., Schroder, K.E., Vanable, P.A. & Gordon, C.M. (2004). HIV risk behavior among psychiatric outpatients: association with psychiatric disorder, substance use disorder, and gender. *Journal of Nervous and Mental Disease.* **192**, 289–96.

Carney, C. & Jones, L. (2006). The influence of type and severity of mental illness on receipt of screening mammography. *Journal of General Internal Medicine.* **21** (10), 1097–104. Carney, C., Jones, L. & Woolson, R. (2006). Medical comorbidity in women and men with schizophrenia: a population-based controlled study. *Journal of General Internal Medicine.* **21**, 1133–37.

Cavanaugh, J., Powell, K., Renwick, O. *et al.* (2012). An outbreak of tuberculosis among adults with mental illness. *American Journal of Psychiatry.* **169**, 569–575.

Chafetz, L., White, M., Collins-Bride, G. & Nickens, J. (2005). The poor general health of the severely mentally ill: impact of schizophrenic diagnosis. *Community Mental Health Journal.* **41**, 169–84.

Chaturvedi, N., McKeigue, P. & Marmot, M. (1994). Relationship of glucose intolerance to coronary risk in Afro-Caribbeans compared with Europeans. *Diabetologia.* **37**, 765–72.

Chaudhury, S., Chandra, S. & Augustine, M. (1994). Prevalence of Australia-Antigen (Hbsag) in institutionalized patients with psychosis. *British Journal of Psychiatry.* **164**, 542–43.

Chengappa, K., Levine, J., Gershon, S. & Kupfer, D. (2000). Lifetime prevalence of substance or alcohol abuse and dependence among subjects with bipolar I and II disorders in a voluntary registry. *Bipolar Disorder.* **2**, 191–195.

Chiu, C., Chen, C., Chen, B. et al. (2010). The time-dependent change of insulin secretion in schizophrenic patients treated with olanzapine. *Progress in Neuro-Psychopharmacology and Biological Psychiatry.* **34** (2010), 866–70.

Chochinov, H., Martens, P.J., Prior, H.J., Fransoo, R. & Burland, E. (2009). The Need To Know Team. Does a diagnosis of schizophrenia reduce rates of mammography screening? A Manitoba population-based study. *Schizophrenia Research.* **113** (1), 95–100.

Cipriani, A., Pretty, H., Hawton, K. et al. (2005). Lithium in the prevention of suicidal behavior and all-cause mortality in patients with mood disorders: a systematic review of randomized trials. *American Journal of Psychiatry.* **162** (10), 1805–19.

Cividini, A., Pistorio, A., Regazzetti, A. et al. (1997). Hepatitis C virus infection among institutionalised psychiatric patients: a regression analysis of indicators of risk. *Journal of Hepatology.* **27**, 455–463.

Cohen, H., Loewenthal, U., Matar, M. & Kotler, M. (2001). Heart rate variability in schizophrenic patients treated with antipsychotic agents. *Harefuah.* **140**, 1142–1147, 1231.

Colton, C. & Manderscheid, R. (2006). Congruencies in increased mortality rates, years of potential life lost, and causes of death among public mental health clients in eightstates. *Preventing Chronic Disease.* **3** (2). http://www.cdc.gov/pcd/issues/2006/apr/05_0180.htm (Accessed 17 December 2014).

Committee for Proprietary Medicinal Products (CPMP) (1997) Point to consider: the assessment of the potential for QT interval prolongation by non cardiovascular medicinal products. http:///www.webcitation.org/query.php?url=http://www.emea.eu.int/pdfs/human/swp/098696en.pdf&refdoi=10.1186/1744-859x-4-1 (Accessed 17 December 2014).

Cookson, J. (2001). Use of antipsychotic drugs and lithium in mania. *British Journal of Psychiatry.* **178** (Suppl 41), S148–56.

Copeland, L., Mortensen, E., Zeber, J. et al. (2007). Pulmonary disease among inpatient decedents: impact of schizophrenia. *Progress in Neuro-Psychopharmacology & Biological Psychiatry.* **31**, 720–26.

Cournos, F., Guido, J., Coomaraswamy, S., Meyer-Bahlburg, H., Sugden, R. & Horwath, E. (1994). Sexual activity and risk of HIV infection among patients with schizophrenia. *American Journal of Psychiatry.* **151**, 228–32.

Cournos, F., McKinnon, M. & Sullivan, G. (2005). Schizophrenia and comorbid Human Immunodeficiency Virus or Hepatitis C Virus. *Journal of Clinical Psychiatry.* **66** (Suppl. 6), 27–33.

Coverdale, J. & Turbott, S. (2000). Risk behaviours for sexually transmitted infections among men with mental disorders. *Psychiatric Services.* **51** (2), 234–38.

Dalton, S., Munk, L., Mellemkjaer, L., Johansen, C. & Mortensen, P. (2003). Schizophrenia and the risk for breast cancer. *Schizophrenia Research.* **62**, 89–92.

Dalton, S.O., Laursen, T.M., Mellemkjaer, L., Johansen, C. & Mortensen, P.B. (2004). Risk for cancer in parents of patients with schizophrenia. *American Journal of Psychiatry.* **161**, 903–908.

Dalton, S., Mellemkjaer, L., Thomassen, L., Mortensen, P. & Johansen, C. (2005). Risk for cancer in a cohort of patients hospitalized for schizophrenia in Denmark, 1969–1993. *Schizophrenia Research.* **75**, 315–24.

Darbàa, J., Minovesb, A., Rojoc, E., Jimenezc, F. & Rejasd, J. (2011). Efficacy of second-generation-antipsychotics in the treatment of negative symptoms of schizophrenia: A meta-analysis of randomized clinical trials. *Revista de Psiquiatría y Salud Mental.* **4** (3), 126–43.

Das, A., Olfson, M., Gameroff, M. et al. (2005). Screening for bipolar disorder in a primary care practice. *Journal of the American Medical Association.* **293**, 956–63.

De Hert, M., Schreurs, V., Vancampfort, D. & Van Winkel, R. (2009). Metabolic syndrome in people with schizophrenia: a review. *World Psychiatry.* **8** (1), 15–22.

De Hert, M., Cohen, D., Bobes, J. *et al.* (2011). Physical illness in patients with severe mental disorders. II. Barriers to care, monitoring and treatment guidelines, plus recommendations at the system and individual level. *World Psychiatry.* **10** (2), 138–51.

Delva, N., Crammer, J., Jarzylo, S. et al. (1989). Osteopenia, pathological fractures, and increased urinary calcium excretion in schizophrenic patients with polydipsia. *Biological Psychiatry.* **26**, 781–93.

DH (Department of Health) (2004). *At Least 5 a Week.* London: The Stationery Office.

DH (Department of Health) (2007a). *NHS Stop Smoking Services and Nicotine Replacement Therapy.* London: The Stationery Office.

DH (Department of Health) (2007b). *Safe. Sensible. Social. The next steps in the National Alcohol Strategy.* London: The Stationery Office.

DH (Department of Health) (2007c). *At least 5 a day.* London: Department of Health.

DH (Department of Health) (2009). *Free NHS Healthcheck.* London: The Stationery Office.

Dougherty, L. & Lister, S. (2004). *The Royal Marsden Hospital Manual of Clinical Nursing Procedures.* 6th edn. London: Blackwell.

Drinkaware (2011). Alcohol Units: your guide to alcohol units and measures. http://www.drinkaware.co.uk/check-the-facts/what-is-alcohol/units-in-common-drinks (Accessed 22 December 2014).

Driscoli, J., Melnick, N., Quinn, F. *et al.* (1978). Psychotropic drugs as potential antitumor agents: a selective screening study. *Cancer Treatment Reports Journal.* **62**, 45–74.

Druss, B., Rosenheck, R., Desai, M. & Perlin, J. (2002). Quality of preventive medical care for patients with mental disorders. *Medical Care.* **40** (2), 129–36.

Dupont, A., Jensen, O., Strömgren, E. & Jablensky, A. (1986). 'Incidence of cancer in patients diagnosed as schizophrenic in Denmark' in G.H. Ten Horn, R. Giel & W.H. Gulbinat (eds.) *Psychiatric Case Registers in Public Health.* Amsterdam: Elsevier.

Einarson, A. & Boskovic, R. (2009). Use and safety of antipsychotic drugs during pregnancy. *Journal of Psychiatric Practice.* **15**, 183–92.

Eldridge, D., Dawber, N. & Gray, R. (2011). A well-being support program for patients with severe mental illness: a service evaluation. *BMC Psychiatry.* **11**, 46. doi:10.1186/1471-244X-11-46.

European Association of Urology (EAU) (2005). *Guidelines on erectile dysfunction.* Arnhem, The Netherlands: EAU.

Fagard, R. (1999). Physical activity in the prevention and rehabilitation of hypertension in the obese. *Medicine and Science in Sports Exercise.* **31**, Suppl 11, S624-630.

Faravelli, C., Guerrini Degl'Innocenti, B., Aiazzi, L. *et al.* (1990). Epidemiology of mood disorders: a community survey in Florence. *Journal of Affective Disorder.* **20**, 135–41.

Feinman, J. & Dunner, D. (1996). The effect of alcohol and substance abuse on the course of bipolar affective disorder. *Journal of Affective Disorder.* **37**, 43–49.

Filik, R., Sipos, A., Kehoe, P. *et al.* (2006). The cardiovascular and respiratory health of people with schizophrenia. *Acta Psychiatrica Scandinavica.* **113**, 298–305.

Fisher, C. & Broderick, W. (2003). Sodium valproate or valproate semisodium: is there a difference in the treatment of bipolar disorder? *The Psychiatrist.* **27**, 446–48.

Fisher, I., Bienskii, A. & Fedorova, I. (1996). Experience in using serological tests in detecting tuberculosis in patients with severe mental pathology. *Problemy Tuberkuleza.* **1**, 19–20.

Foulds, J., Steinberg, M., Richardson, D. *et al.* (2006). Factors associated with quitting smoking at a tobacco dependence treatment clinic. *American Journal of Health Behavior.* **30**, 400–412.

Friedlander, A. & Marder, S. (2002). The psychopathology, medical management and dental implications of schizophrenia. *Journal of the American Dental Association.* **133**, 603–610.

Frye, M., Altshuler, L., McElroy, S., Suppes, T., Keck, P., Denicoff, K. *et al.* (2003). Gender differences in prevalence, risk, and clinical correlates of alcoholism comorbidity in bipolar disorder. *American Journal of Psychiatry.* **160**, 883–89.

Garcia-Unzueta, M., Herran, A., Sierra-Biddle, D., Amado, J., Vazquez-Barquero, J. & Alvarez, C. (2003). Alterations of liver function test in patients treated with antipsychotics. *Journal of Clinical Laboratory Analysis.* **17**, 216–18.

Geddes, J., Burgess, S., Hawton, K. *et al.* (2004). Long-term lithium therapy for bipolar disorder: systematic review and meta-analysis of randomized controlled trials. *American Journal of Psychiatry.* **161** (2), 217–22.

Goldacre, M., Kurina, L., Wotton, C., Yeates, D. & Seagroat, V. (2005). Schizophrenia and cancer: an epidemiological study. *British Journal of Psychiatry.* **187**, 334–38.

Goldney, R., Phillips, P., Fisher, L. & Wilson, D. (2004). Diabetes, depression, and quality of life: a population study. *Diabetes Care.* **27**, 1066–70.

Goldney, R., Fisher, L., Grande, E. *et al.* (2005). Bipolar I and II disorders in a random and representative Australian population. *Australia and New Zealand Journal of Psychiatry.* **39**, 726–29.

Goodwin, G. (2009). Evidence-based guidelines for treating bipolar disorder: revised second edition – recommendations from the British Association for Psychopharmacology. *Journal of Psychopharmacology.* **23**, (4), 346–88.

Gordon, C., Carey, M., Carey, K. *et al.* (1999). Understanding HIV-related risk among persons with a severe and persistent mental illness: insights from a qualitative inquiry. *Journal of Nervous and Mental Disease.* **187**, 208–16.

Gough, S. & Peveler, R. (2004). Diabetes and its prevention: pragmatic solutions for people with schizophrenia. *British Journal of Psychiatry.* **184**, (Suppl. 47), s106–s111.

Grant, B., Stinson, F., Hasin, D., Dawson, D., Chou, S., Ruan, W. *et al.* (2005). Prevalence, correlates, and comorbidity of bipolar I disorder and axis I and II disorders: results from the National Epidemiologic Survey on Alcohol and Related Conditions. *Journal of Clinical Psychiatry.* **66**, 1205–215.

Gray, R., Brewin, E., Noak, J., Wyke-Joseph, J. & Sonik, B. (2002). A review of the literature on HIV infection and schizophrenia: implications for research, policy and clinical practice. *Journal of Psychiatric and Mental Health Nursing.* **9**, 405–409.

Grigsby, A., Anderson, R., Freedland, K. *et al.* (2002). Prevalence of anxiety in adults with diabetes: a systematic review. *Journal of Psychosomatic Research.* **53**, 1053–60.

Grinshpoon, A., Barchana, M., Ponizovsky, A. *et al.* (2005). Cancer in schizophrenia: is the risk higher or lower? *Schizophrenia Research.* **73**, 333–41.

Guggar, J. (2011). Antipsychotic pharmacotherapy and orthostatic hypotension: identification and management. *CNS Drugs.* **25**, (8), 659–71.

Gulbinat, W., Dupont, A., Jablensky, A. *et al.* (1992). Cancer incidence of schizophrenic patients. Results of record linkage studies in three countries. *British Journal of Psychiatry.* Suppl 18, 75–83.

Gupta, S., Masand, P., Kaplan, D. *et al.* (1997). The relationship between schizophrenia and irritable bowel syndrome (IBS). *Schizophrenia Research.* **23**, (3), 265–8.

Haddad, P., Hellewell, J. & Wieck, A. (2001). Antipsychotic induced hyperprolactinaemia: a series of illustrative case reports. *Journal of Psychopharmacology.* **15**, (4), 293–95.

Halbreich, U., Kinon, B., Gilmore, J. & Kahn, L. (2003). Elevated prolactin levels in patients with schizophrenia: mechanisms and related adverse effects. *Psychoneuroendocrinology.* **28**, (1), 53–67.

Halbreich, U. & Palter, S. (1996). Accelerated osteoporosis in psychiatric patients: possible pathophysiological processes. *Schizophrenia Bulletin.* **22**, 447–54.

Halbreich, U., Rojansky, N., Palter, S. *et al.* (1995). Decreased bone mineral density in medicated psychiatric patients. *Psychosomatic Medicine.* **57**, 485–91.

Hanssens, L. *et al.* (2006). APA Annual Meeting. Poster NR361.

Hardy, S. & Gray, R. (2012). *The Primary Care Guide to Mental Health*. Keswick: M&K Update.

Harrison & Weinberger (2005). Schizophrenia genes, gene expression, and neuropathology: on the matter of their convergence. *Molecular Psychiatry.* **10**, (1), 40–68.

Hartz, S., Pato, C., Medeiros, H. *et al.* (2014). Comorbidity of severe psychotic disorders with measures of substance use. *JAMA Psychiatry.* **71**, (3), 248–54.

Health and Social Care Information Centre (2010). *Health Survey for England - 2009, Trend Tables*. London: The NHS Information Centre for Health and Social Care.

Henderson, D., Borba, C., Daley, T., Boxill, R., Nguyen, D., Culhane, M., Louie, P., Cather, C., Eden Evins, A., Freudenreich, O., Taber, S. & Goff, D. (2006). Dietary intake profile of patients with schizophrenia. *Annals of Clinical Psychiatry.* **18**, (2), 99–105.

Hennekens, C.H., Hennekens, A.R., Hollar, D. *et al.* (2005). Schizophrenia and increased risks of cardiovascular disease. *American Heart Journal.* **150**, 1115–121.

Henquet, C., Murray, R., Linszen, D. & van Os, J. (2005). The environment and schizophrenia: the role of cannabis use. *Schizophrenia Bulletin.* **31** (3), 608–12.

Himelhoch, S., Lehman, A., Kreyenbuhl, J. *et al.* (2004). Prevalence of chronic obstructive pulmonary disease among those with serious mental illness. *American Journal of Psychiatry.* **161**, 2317–19.

Hippisley-Cox, J., Vinogradova, Y., Coupland, C. *et al.* (2007). Risk of malignancy in patients with schizophrenia or bipolar disorder: nested case-control study. *Archives of General Psychiatry.* **64**, 1368–76.

Hofstetter, J., Lysaker, P. & Mayeda, A. (2005). Quality of sleep in patients with schizophrenia is associated with quality of life and coping. *BMC Psychiatry.* **5**, 13.

Holt, R. & Peveler, R. (2005). Association between antipsychotic drugs and diabetes. *Diabetes, Obesity and Metabolism.* **8**, 125–35.

Holt, R. & Peveler, R. (2009). Obesity, serious mental illness and antipsychotic drugs. *Diabetes, Obesity and Metabolism.* **11** (7), 665–79.

Holt, R. & Peveler, R. (2010). Diabetes and cardiovascular risk in severe mental illness: a missed opportunity and challenge for the future. *Practical Diabetes International.* **27**, 79–84.

Holt, R. & Peveler, R. (2011). Antipsychotic and hyperprolactinaemia: mechanisms, consequences and management. *Clinical Endocrinology.* **74**, 141–47.

Huang, H., Matevossian, A., Whittle, C. *et al.* (2007). Prefrontal dysfunction in schizophrenia involves mixed-lineage leukemia 1-regulated histone methylation at GABAergic gene promoters. Information Services Publications and Presentations. Paper 34. http://escholarship.umassmed.edu/infoservices/34 (Accessed 22 December 2014).

Hummer, M., Malik, P., Gasser, R. et al. (2005). Osteoporosis in patients with schizophrenia. *American Journal of Psychiatry.* **162**, 162–67.

Jeste, D., Dgladsjo, J., Lindamer, L. *et al.* (1996). Medical comorbidity in schizophrenia. *Schizophrenia Bulletin.* 22, 413–20.

Johnson, J., Ratner, P., Malchy, L. *et al.* (2010). Gender-specific profiles of tobacco use among non-institutionalised people with serious mental illness. *BMC Psychiatry.* **10**, 101.

Jones, I. & Smith, S. (2009). Puerperal psychosis: identifying and caring for women at risk. *Advances in Psychiatric Treatment.* **15**, 411–18.

Kalichman, S., Sikkema, K., Kelly, J. *et al.* (1994). Factors associated with risk for HIV infection among chronic mentally ill adults. *American Journal of Psychiatry.* **15**, 221–27.

Kalkan, A., Ozdarendeli, A., Bulut, Y. *et al.* (2005). Prevalence and genotypic distribution of hepatitis GB-C/HG and TT viruses in blood donors, mentally retarded children and four groups of patients in eastern Anatolia, Turkey. *Japanese Journal of Infectious Diseases.* **58**, 222–27.

Kantor, M., Cullinane, E., Sady, S., Herbert, P. & Thompson, P. (1987). Exercise acutely increases HDL-cholesterol and lipoprotein lipase activity in trained and untrained men. *Metabolism.* **36**, 188–92.

Kapur, S., Agid, O., Mizrahi, R. & Li, M. (2006). How antipsychotics work – from receptors to reality. *NeuroRx.* **3** (1), 10–21.

Kasperek-Zimowska, B., Brodniak, W.A. & Sarol-Kulka, A. (2008). Sexual disorders in schizophrenia – overview of research literature. *Psychiatria Polska.* **42**, 97–104.

Keely, E., Reiss, J., Drinkwater, D. & Faiman, C. (1997). Bone mineral density, sex hormones, and long-term use of neuroleptic agents in men. *Endocrine Practice.* **3**, 209–213.

Kenkre, A. & Spadigam, A. (2000). Oral health and treatment needs in institutionalized psychiatric inpatients in India. *Indian Journal of Dental Research.* **11**, 5–11.

Kesaniemi, Y., Danforth, E., Jensen, M., Kopelman, P., Lefebvre, P. & Reeder, B. (2001). Consensus statement. Dose response issues concerning physical activity and health: an evidence-based symposium. *Medicine & Science in Sports & Exercise.* **33** (Suppl 6), S351–8.

Kessler, R., Crum, R., Warner, L., Nelson, C., Schulenberg, J. & Anthony, J. (1997). Lifetime co-occurrence of DSM-III-R alcohol abuse and dependence with other psychiatric disorders in the National Comorbidity Survey. *Archives of General Psychiatry.* **54**, 313–21.

Kishimoto, T., Watanabe, K., Takeuchi, H. et al. (2005). Bone mineral density measurement in female inpatients with schizophrenia. *Schizophrenia Research.* **77**, 113–15.

Kudoh, A., Ishihara, H. & Matsuki, A. (1999). Pituitary-adrenal and parasympathetic function in chronic schizophrenic patients with postoperative ileus or hypotension. *Neuropsychobiology.* **39**, 125–30.

Lacro, J.P., Dunn, L.B., Dolder, C.R., Leckband, S.G. & Jeste, D.V. (2002). Prevalence of and risk factors for medication non-adherence in patients with schizophrenia: a comprehensive review of the literature. *The Journal of Clinical Psychiatry.* **63**, 892–909.

Lavin, M., Siris, S. & Mason, S. (1996). What is the clinical importance of cigarette smoking in schizophrenia? *American Journal of Addictions.* **5**, 189–208.

Lawrence, D., Holman, C., Jablensky, A., Threlfall, T. & Fuller, S. (2000). Excess cancer mortality in Western Australian psychiatric patients due to higher case fatality rates. *Acta Psychiatrica Scandinavica.* **101**, 382–88.

Leucht, S., Tardy, M., Komossa, K., Heres, S., Kissling, W., Salanti, G. & Davis, J.M. (2012) Antipsychotic drugs versus placebo for relapse prevention in schizophrenia: a systematic review and meta-analysis. *Lancet.* **379**, 2063–71.

Leucht, S., Burkard, T., Henderson, J., Maj, M. & Sartorius, N. (2007). Physical illness and schizophrenia: a review of the literature. *Acta Psychiatrica Scandinavica.* **116** (5), 317–33.

Lewis, S., Jagger, R. & Treasure, E. (2001). The oral health of psychiatric in-patients in South Wales. *Special Care Dentistry.* **21**, 182–86.

Lichtermann, D., Ekelund, J., Pukkala, E., Tanskanen, A. & Lonnqvist, J. (2001). Incidence of cancer among persons with schizophrenia and their relatives. *Archives of General Psychiatry.* **58**, 573–78.

Lip, G., Barnett, A., Bradbury, A., Cappuccio, F., Gill, P., Hughes, E., Imray, C., Jolly, K. & Patel, K. (2007). Ethnicity and cardiovascular disease prevention in the United Kingdom: a practical approach to management. *Journal of Human Hypertension.* **21** (3), 183–211.

Liperoti, R., Gambassi, G., Lapane, K. *et al.* (2005). Conventional and atypical antipsychotics and the risk of hospitalization for ventricular arrhythmias or cardiac arrest. *Archives of Internal Medicine.* **165**, 696–701.

Liu-Seifert, H., Kinon, B., Ahl, J. & Lamberson, S. (2004). Osteopenia associated with increased prolactin and aging in psychiatric patients treated with prolactin-elevating antipsychotics. *Annals of the New York Academy of Sciences.* **1032**, 297–98.

Mantere, O., Suominen, K., Leppamaki, S. *et al.* (2004). The clinical characteristics of DSM-IV bipolar I and II disorders: baseline findings from the Jorvi Bipolar Study (JoBS). *Bipolar Disorders.* **6**, 395–405.

Manu, P., Correll, C.U., van Winkel, R. *et al.* (2012). Prediabetes in patients treated with antipsychotic drugs. *Journal of Clinical Psychiatry.* **73** (4), 460–66.

Marmota, M. (1983). Alcohol and Coronary Heart Disease. *International Journal of Epidemiology.* **30** (4), 724–29.

Matsui-Sakata, A., Ohtani, H. & Sawad, Y. (2005). Receptor occupancy-based analysis of the contributions of various receptors to antipsychotics-induced weight gain and diabetes mellitus. *Drug Metabolism and Pharmacokinetics.* **20** (5), 368–78.

McCreadie, R. (2003). Diet, smoking and cardiovascular disease risk in people with schizophrenia. Descriptive study. *British Journal of Psychiatry.* **183**, 534–39.

McCreadie, R., Stevens, H., Henderson, J. et al. (2004). The dental health of people with schizophrenia. *Acta Psychiatrica Scandinavica.* **110**, 306–310.

McCreadie, R., Kelly, C., Connolly, M. *et al.* (2005). Dietary improvement in people with schizophrenia. *The British Journal of Psychiatry.* **187**, 346–51.

Mcdonald, S., Halliday, J., Macewan, T. *et al.* (2003). Nithsdale schizophrenia surveys 24: sexual dysfunction. Case-control study. *British Journal of Psychiatry.* **182**, 50–56.

McGahuey, C., Gelenberg, A., Laukes, C., Moreno, F., Delgado, P., McKnight, K. & Manber, R. (2000). The Arizona Sexual Experience Scale (ASEX): reliability and validity. *Journal of Sex and Marital Therapy.* **26** (1), 25–40.

McKeigue, P., Shah, B. & Marmot, M. (1991). Relation of central obesity and insulin resistance with high diabetes prevalence and cardiovascular risk in South Asians. *Lancet.* **337**, 382–86.

Meaney, A., Smith, S., Howes, O., O'Brien, M., Murray, R. & O'Keane, V. (2004). Effects of long-term prolactin-raising antipsychotic medication on bone mineral density in patients with schizophrenia. *British Journal of Psychiatry.* **184**, 503–508.

Melle, I., Johannesen, J., Friis, S., Haahr, U., Joa, I., Larsen, T., Opjordsmoen Bjørn, R., Rund, B., Simonsen, E., Vaglum, P. & McGlashan, T. (2006). Early detection of the first episode of schizophrenia and suicidal behavior. *American Journal of Psychiatry.* **163**, 800–804.

Meltzer, H., Gill, B., Pettigrew, M. *et al.* (1996). *OPCS Survey of Psychiatric Morbidity in Great Britain. Report 3: Economic activity and social functioning of adults with psychiatric disorders.* London: The Stationery Office.

Mercuro, G., Deidda, M., Piras, A., Dessalvi, C., Maffei, S. & Rosano, G. (2010). Gender determinants of cardiovascular risk factors and diseases. *Journal of Cardiovascular Medicine.* **11**, 3, 207–20.

Mitchell, A., Vancampfort, D., Sweers, K. *et al.* (2011). Prevalence of metabolic syndrome and metabolic abnormalities in schizophrenia and related disorders – a systematic review and meta-analysis. *Schizophrenia Bulletin.* [Epub ahead of print]

Morken, G., Widen, J. & Grawe, R. (2008). Non-compliance to antipsychotic medications, relapse and rehospitalization in recent-onset schizophrenia. *BMC Psychiatry.* **8**, 32.

Morrish, N., Wang, S., Stevens, L., Fuller, J. & Keen, H. (2001). Mortality and causes of death in the WHO Multinational Study of Vascular Disease in Diabetes. *Diabetologia.* **44**, Suppl 2 S14–S21.

Mortensen, P. (1989). The incidence of cancer in schizophrenic patients. *Journal of Epidemiological Community Health.* **43**, 43–47.

Mortensen, P. (1992). Neuroleptic medication and reduced risk of prostate cancer in schizophrenic patients. *Acta Psychiatrica Scandinavica.* **85**, 390–93.

Mortensen, P. (1994). The occurrence of cancer in first admitted schizophrenic patients. *Schizophrenia Research.* **12**, 185–94.

Mueser, K. & McGurk, S. (2004). Schizophrenia. *The Lancet.* **363** (9426), 2063–72.

Nakamura, Y., Koh, M., Miyoshi, E. *et al.* (2004). High prevalence of the hepatitis C virus infection among the inpatients of schizophrenia and psychoactive substance abuse in Japan. *Progress in Neuro-Psychopharmacology & Biological Psychiatry.* **28**, 591–97.

Nakane, Y. & Ohta, Y. (1986). 'The example of linkage with a cancer register' in G.H. Ten Horn, R. Giel, W.H. Gulbinat (eds). *Psychiatric Case Registers in Public Health.* Amsterdam: Elsevier.

Nasrallah, H. (2003). A review of the effect of atypical antipsychotics on weight. *Psychoneuroendocrinology.* **28** (1), 83–96.

National Obesity Forum (2011). Waist circumference. http:///www.nationalobesityforum.org.uk/training-resource-for-healthcare-professionals-mainmenu-133/assessment-mainmenu-168/171-waist-circumference.html (Accessed 22 December 2014).

National Statistics, Health Statistics Quarterly 07, Autumn 2000 http://www.ons.gov.uk/ons/search/index.html?pageSize=50&sortBy=none&sortDirection=none&newquery=2000+autumn+quarterly (Accessed 30 December 2014).

Newcomer, J., Haupt, D., Fucetola, R., Melson, A., Schweiger, J., Cooper, B. & Selke, G. (2002). Abnormalities in glucose regulation during antipsychotic treatment of schizophrenia. *Archives of General Psychiatry.* **59**, 337–45.

NHS Cancer Screening Programmes (2009a). NHS Cervical Screening Programme. http://www.cancerscreening.nhs.uk/cervical/index.html#eligible (Accessed 22 December 2014).

NHS Cancer Screening Programmes (2009b). NHS Bowel Cancer Screening Programme. http://www.cancerscreening.nhs.uk/bowel/#gps-involved (Accessed 22 December 2014).

NHS Choices (2009). Benefits of going smokefree. http://smokefree.nhs.uk/why-go-smokefree/benefits-of-going-smokefree/ (Accessed 22 December 2014).

NHS Choices (2013). Preventing dehydration. http://www.nhs.uk/conditions/dehydration/pages/prevention.aspx (Accessed 22 December 2014).

NHS Information Centre (2010). *Statistics on Alcohol: England, 2010.* NHS Information Centre. http://www.hscic.gov.uk/catalogue/PUB00135/alco-eng-2010-rep.pdf (Accessed 30 December 2014).

NICE (National Institute for Health and Clinical Excellence) (2004a). *CG19 Dental Recall. Recall interval between routine dental examinations.* London: NICE.

NICE (National Institute for Health and Clinical Excellence) (2004b). *Improving Outcomes in Colorectal Cancers.* http://guidance.nice.org.uk/CSGCC (Accessed 22 December 2014).

NICE (National Institute for Health and Clinical Excellence) (2006). *The management of bipolar disorder in adults, children and adolescents, in primary and secondary care NICE clinical guideline 38.* London: NICE.

NICE (National Institute for Health and Clinical Excellence) (2014). *Lipid Modification.* http://www.nice.org.uk/guidance/cg181 (Accessed 30 December 2014).

NICE (National Institute for Health and Clinical Excellence) (2011). *Clinical management of primary hypertension in adults.* http://www.nice.org.uk/guidance/cg127/resources/guidance-hypertension-pdf (Accessed 30 December 2014).

NICE (National Institute for Health and Clinical Excellence) (2014). *Psychosis and schizophrenia in adults. National Collaborating Centre for Mental Health commissioned by the National Institute for Health and Care Excellence.* London: NICE.

Nordestgaard, B., Benn, M., Schnohr, P. & Tybjærg-Hansen, A. (2007). Nonfasting triglycerides and risk of myocardial infarction, ischemic heart disease, and death in men and women. *Journal of the American Medical Association.* **298** (3), 299–308.

NWMHP (Norfolk and Waveney Mental Health Partnership NHS Trust) (2013). NWMHP Pharmacy Medicine Information: caffeine. http://www.choiceandmedication.org/nsft/medications/112/ (Accessed 22 December 2014).

Ohta, Y., Nakane, Y., Mine, M. et al. (1988). The epidemiological study of physical morbidity in schizophrenics–2. Association between schizophrenia and incidence of tuberculosis. *Japanese Journal of Psychiatry and Neurology.* **42**, 41–47.

O'Keane, V. & Meaney, A. (2005). Antipsychotic drugs: a new risk factor for osteoporosis in young women with schizophrenia? *Journal of Clinical Psychopharmacology.* **25**, 26–31.

Osborn, D., Nazareth, I. & King, M. (2006). Risk for coronary heart disease in people with severe mental illness. *The British Journal of Psychiatry.* **188**, 271–77.

Osborn, D., Levy, G., Nazareth, I., Petersen, I., Islam, A. & King, M. (2007). Relative risk of cardiovascular and cancer mortality in people with severe mental illness from the United Kingdom's General Practice Research Database. *Archives of General Psychiatry.* **64** (2), 242–49.

Osborn, D., Limburg, H., Walters, K., Petersen, I., King, M., Green, J., Watson, J. & Nazareth, I. (2013). Relative incidence of common cancers in people with severe mental illness. Cohort study in the United Kingdom THIN primary care database. *Schizophrenia Research.* **43** (1), 44–49.

Othman, S., Kadir, K., Hassan, J., Hong, G., Singh, B. & Raman, N. (1994). High prevalence of thyroid function test abnormalities in chronic schizophrenia. *Australian and New Zealand Journal of Psychiatry.* **28** (4), 620–24.

Oud, M. & Meyboom-de Jong, B. (2009). Somatic diseases in patients with schizophrenia in general practice: their prevalence and health care. *BMC Family Practice.* **10** (32). doi:10.1186/1471-2296-10-32.

Palmer, B., McClure, S. & Jeste, D. (2001). Schizophrenia in late life: Findings challenge traditional concepts. *Harvard Review of Psychiatry.* **3**, 51–58.

Pantelis, C. & Lambert, T. (2003). Managing patients with 'treatment-resistant' schizophrenia. *Medical Journal of Australia.* **178** (suppl.) S62–S66.

Parikh, P., McDaniel, M., Ashen, D. et al. (2005). Diets and cardiovascular disease: an evidence-based assessment. *American College of Cardiology.* **45** (9), 1379–87.

Patient UK (2005). Polyuria. http://www.patient.co.uk/doctor/Polyuria.htm (Accessed 22 December 2014).

Patient UK (2006). Neuroleptic Malignant Syndrome. http://www.patient.co.uk/showdoc/40025090/ (Accessed 22 December 2014).

Patient UK (2007). Breast lumps and breast examination. http:///www.patient.co.uk/showdoc/40000260 (Accessed 22 December 2014).

Patient UK (2008). Oliguria. http://www.patient.co.uk/doctor/Oliguria.htm (Accessed 22 December 2014).

Peet, M. (2004). International variations in the outcome of schizophrenia and the prevalence of depression in relation to national dietary practices: an ecological analysis. *The British Journal of Psychiatry.* **184**, 404–408.

Peto, J., Gilham, C., Fletcher, O. & Matthews, F. (2004). The cervical cancer epidemic that screening has prevented in the UK. *The Lancet.* **364**, 249–56.

Peveler, R., Branford, D., Citrome, L. *et al.* (2008). Antipsychotics and hyperprolactinaemia: Clinical recommendations. *Journal of Psychopharmacology.* **22** (2), 98–103.

Phelan, M., Stradins, L. & Morrison, S. (2001). Physical health of people with severe mental illness. *British Medical Journal.* **322**, 443–44.

Pilling, S., Bebbington, P., Kuipers, E. *et al.* (2002). Psychological treatment in schizophrenia: I. Metaanalysis of family intervention and cognitive behaviour therapy. *Psychological Medicine.* **32**, 763–82.

Pini, S., de Queiroz, V., Pagnin, D. *et al.* (2005). Prevalence and burden of bipolar disorders in European countries. European *Neuropsychopharmacology.* 425–34.

Poirer, P., Giles, T., Bray, G. *et al.* (2006). Obesity and cardiovascular disease. Pathophysiology, evaluation, and effect of weight loss. *Arteriosclerosis, Thrombosis, and Vascular Biology.* **26**, 968–76.

Priebe, S., Yeeles, K., Bremner, S., Lauber, C., Eldridge, S., Ashby, D. *et al.* (2013). Effectiveness of financial incentives to improve adherence to maintenance treatment with antipsychotics: cluster randomised controlled trial. *British Medical Journal.* **347**, f5847.

Prince, D., Walkup, J., Akincigil, A. *et al.* (2012). Serious mental illness and risk of new HIV/AIDS diagnoses: an analysis of medicaid beneficiaries in eight states. *Psychiatric Services.* **63** (10), 1261–62.

Prochaska, J.O., Norcross, J.C. & Diclemente, C.C. (1994). *Changing for Good.* New York: Avon Books.

Ray, W., Meredith, S., Thapa, P. *et al.* (2001). Antipsychotics and the risk of sudden cardiac death. *Archives of General Psychiatry.* **58**, 1161–1167.

Regier, D., Farmer, M., Rae, D., Locke, B., Keith, S., Judd, L. *et al.* (1990). Comorbidity of mental disorders with alcohol and other drug abuse. Results from the Epidemiologic Catchment Area (ECA) Study. *Journal of the American Medical Association.* **264**, 2511–18.

Rethink (2008). Antipsychotic Medication. https://www.rethink.org/diagnosis-treatment/medications/antipsychotics (Accessed 30 December 2014).

Rimm, E., Giovannucci, E., Willett, W. *et al.* (1991). Prospective study of alcohol consumption and risk of coronary disease in men. *The Lancet.* **338** (8765), 464–68.

Robson, D. & Gray, R. (2007). Serious mental illness and physical health problems: a discussion paper. *International Journal of Nursing Studies.* **44**, 457–66.

Rosenberg, S., Goodman, L., Osher, F. *et al.* (2001). Prevalence of HIV, hepatitis B, and hepatitis C in people with severe mental illness. *American Journal of Public Health.* **91**, 31–37.

Rosenberg, S., Drake, R., Brunette, M. *et al.* (2005). Hepatitis C virus and HIV co-infection in people with severe mental illness and substance use disorders. *AIDS.* Suppl 3 S26–33.

Rosenheck, R., Leslie, D., Keefe, R., McEvoy, J., Swartz, M., Perkins, D., Stroup, S., Hsiao, J. & Lieberman, J. CATIE Study Investigators Group (2006). Barriers to employment for people with schizophrenia. *American Journal of Psychiatry.* **163** 411–17.

Royal College of Psychiatrists and Royal College of General Practitioners (2010). Pharmacy Guidance on smoking and mental health. http://www.rcpsych.ac.uk/pdf/Pharmacy_%20guidance%20for%20smoking%20and%20mental%20health%20Feb%202010.pdf (Accessed 22 December 2014).

Saha, S., Chant, D. & Mcgrath, J. (2008). Meta-analyses of the incidence and prevalence of schizophrenia: conceptual and methodological issues. *International Journal of Methods in Psychiatric Research.* **17**, 55–61.

Said, W., Saleh, R. & Jumaian, N. (2001). Prevalence of hepatitis B virus among chronic schizophrenia patients. *Eastern Mediterranean Health Journal.* **7**, 526–530.

Sasieni, P., Cuzick, J. & Lynch-Farmery, E. (1996). Estimating the efficacy of screening by auditing smear histories of women with and without cervical cancer. The National Co-ordinating Network for Cervical Screening Working Group. *British Journal of Cancer.* **73** (8), 1001–1005.

Schulz, M., Gray, R., Spiekermann, A., Abderhalden, C., Behrens, J. & Driessen, M. (2013). Adherence therapy following an acute episode of schizophrenia: a multi-centre randomised controlled trial. *Schizophrenia Research.* **146**, 1–3.

Scottish Intercollegiate Guidelines Network (SIGN) (2013). SIGN 131 – The management of schizophrenia. http://www.sign.ac.uk/guidelines/fulltext/131/index.html (Accessed 22 December 2014).

Smith, S., O'Keane, V. & Murray, R. (2002). Sexual dysfunction in patients taking conventional antipsychotic medication. *British Journal of Psychiatry.* **181**, 49–55.

Society of Chiropodists and Podiatrists (2007). *Professional care.* London: Society of Chiropodists and Podiatrists.

Sokal, J., Messias, E., Dickerson, F. *et al.* (2004). Comorbidity of medical illnesses among adults with serious mental illness who are receiving community psychiatric services. *Journal of Nervous and Mental Disease.* **192**, 421–27.

Szadoczky, E., Papp, Z., Vitrai, J. *et al.* (1998). The prevalence of major depressive and bipolar disorders in Hungary. Results from a national epidemiologic survey. *Journal of Affective Disorders.* **50**, 153–62.

Tang, W., Sun, F., Ungvari, G. & O'Donnell, D. (2004). Oral health of psychiatric in-patients in Hong Kong. *International Journal of Social Psychiatry.* **50**, 186–91.

Taylor, D., Paton, C. & Kerwin, R. (2007). *Maudsley Prescribing Guidelines.* 9th edn. Informa Healthcare.

Taylor, R., Keil, D., Gold, E., Williams, S. & Goulding, A. (1998). Body mass index, waist girth, and regional adiposity in women: evaluation using receiver operating characteristic curves. *American Journal of Clinical Nutrition.* **67**, 44–49.

Teixeira, J., Rebelo, D., Simões do Couto, F. & Figueira, M. (2009). Requisition of blood analysis for patients with schizophrenia upon acute admission. *European Psychiatry.* **24** (1), s1200.

ten Have, M., Vollebergh, W., Bijl, R. *et al.* (2002). Bipolar disorder in the general population in the Netherlands (prevalence, consequences and care utilisation): results from the Netherlands Mental Health Survey and Incidence Study (NEMESIS). *Journal of Affective Disorders.* **68**, 203–213.

Thakore, J., Mann, J., Vlahos, I., Martin, A. & Reznek, R. (2002). Increased visceral fat distribution in drug-naive and drug-free patients with schizophrenia. *International Journal of Obesity and Related Metabolic Disorders.* (1) 137–41.

Thomas, A., Lavrentzou, E., Karouzos, C. *et al.* (1996). Factors which influence the oral condition of chronic schizophrenia patients. *Specialist Care Dentistry.* **16**, 84–86.

Thornicroft, G. (2011). Physical health disparities and mental illness: the scandal of premature mortality. *British Journal of Psychiatry.* **199**, 441–42.

Tiihonen, J., Lönnqvist, J., Wahlbeck, K. *et al.* (2009). 11 year follow up of mortality in patients with schizophrenia: a population based cohort study. *The Lancet.* **374**, 620–7.

Trixler, M., Gati, A., Fekete, S. *et al.* (2005). Use of antipsychotics in the management of schizophrenia during pregnancy. *Drugs.* **65**, 1193–206.

Tsuang, M., Stone, W. & Faraone, S. (2001). Genes, environment and schizophrenia. *The British Journal of Psychiatry.* **178**, s18–s24.

Vancampfort, D., Vansteelandt, K., Correll, C.U., *et al.* (2013). Prevalence of metabolic syndrome and metabolic abnormalities in bipolar disorders – a systematic review and meta-analysis. *American Journal of Psychiatry.* doi: 10.1176/appi.ajp.2012.12050620. [Epub ahead of print]

Van Rossum, J. (1967). 'Neuropsychopharmacology, Proceedings Fifth Collegium Internationale Neuropsychopharmacologicum' in H. Brill, J. Cole, P. Deniker, H. Hippius, P.B. Bradley (eds) Taylor, D., Paton, C. & Kerwin, R. (2007). *Maudsley Prescribing Guidelines.* 9th edn. Informa Healthcare. *Neuropsychopharmacology Amsterdam:* Excerpta Medica. 321–29.

Vázquez, M. & Beltrán, T. (2007). Neuroleptic malignant syndrome: Possible relationship between Neuroleptic Treatment and Smoking Cessation. *European Journal of Psychiatry.* **21**, 4.

Velasco, E., Machuca, G., Martinez-Sahuquillo, A., Rios, V., Lacalle, J. & Bullon, P. (1997). Dental health among institutionalized psychiatric patients in Spain. *Specialist Care Dentistry.* **17**, 203–206.

Velasco-Ortega, E., Monsalve-Guil, L., Velasco-Ponferrada, C., Medel-Soteras, R. & Segura-Egea, J. (2005). Temporomandibular disorders among schizophrenic patients. A case-control study. *Medicina Oral Patologia Oral y Cirugia Bucal.* **10**, 315–22.

Velligan, D.I., Diamond, P.M., Mintz, J., Maples, N., Li, X., Zeber, J., Ereshefsky, L., Lam, Y.W., Castillo, D. & Miller, A.L. (2008). The use of individually tailored environmental supports to improve medication adherence and outcomes in schizophrenia. *Schizophrenia Bulletin.* **34** (3), 483–93.

Vogel, R. (2002). Alcohol, heart disease, and mortality: a review. *Reviews in Cardiovascular Medicine.* **3** (1), 7–13.

Wahlbeck, K., Westman, J., Nordentoft, M. *et al.* (2011). Outcomes of Nordic mental health systems: life expectancy of persons with mental disorders. *British Journal of Psychiatry.* **199** 453–58.

Walsh, T., McClellan, J., McCarthy, S. *et al.* (2008). Rare structuralvariants disrupt multiple genes in neurodevelopmental pathwaysin schizophrenia. *Science.* **320**, 539–43.

Wang, T., Pencina, M., Booth, S. *et al.* (2008). Vitamin D deficiency and risk of cardiovascular disease. *Circulation.* **117**, 503–511.

Werneke, U., Horn, O., Maryon-Davis, A. *et al.* (2006). Uptake of screening for breast cancer in patients with mental health problems. *Journal of Epidemiological Community Health.* **60** (7), 600–605.

White, J. (2010). Evaluation of the serious mental illness Health Improvement Profile [HIP]: The HIP 100. *16th International Network for Psychiatric Nursing Research (NPNR) Conference: Collaborative research and partnership working.* 23 September 2010, Wadham College, Oxford.

WHO (World Health Organization) (2006). Updated 2009http://apps.who.int/bmi/index.jsp?introPage=intro_3.html (Accessed 30 December 2014).

WHO (World Health Organization) (2011). Cardiovascular disease. http://www.who.int/mediacentre/factsheets/fs317/en/index.html (Accessed 23 December 2014).

Williams, G. & Pickup, J. (2004). *Handbook of Diabetes.* 3rd edn. London: Blackwell Publishing.

Williams, R., Hunt, S., Heiss, G. *et al.* (2001). Usefulness of cardiovascular family history data for population-based preventive medicine and medical research (The Health Family Tree Study and the NHLBI Family Heart Study). *The American Journal of Cardiology.* **87** (2), 129–35.

Williams, B., Poulter, N., Brown, M. *et al.* (2004). Guidelines for management of hypertension: report of the fourth working party of the British Hypertension Society, 2004—BHS IV. *Journal of Human Hypertension.* **18**, 139–85.

Wilson, P., D'Agostino, R., Sullivan, L., Parise, H. & Kannel, W. (2002). Overweight and obesity as determinants of cardiovascular risk: The Framingham experience. *Archives of International Medicine.* **162**, 1867–72. doi: 10.1001/archinte.162.16.1867.

Wood, D., De Backer, G., Faergeman, O., Graham, I., Mancia, G. & Pyörälä, K. (1998). Prevention of coronary heart disease in clinical practice. Recommendations of the second Joint Task Force of European and other Societies on coronary prevention. *Journal of Hypertension.* **16** (10), 1407–414.

World Heart Federation. (2012) Cardiovascular disease risk factors. http://www.world-heart-federation.org/cardiovascular-health/cardiovascular-disease-risk-factors/ (Accessed 30 December 2014).

Worrel, J.A., Marken, P.A., Beckman, S.E. & Ruehter, V.L. (2000). Atypical antipsychotic agents: a critical review. *American Journal of Health System Pharmacy.* **57**, 238–55.

Zeenreich, A., Gochstein, B., Grinshpoon, A., Miron, M., Rosenman, J. & Ben Dov, I. (1998). Recurrent tuberculosis in a psychiatric hospital, recurrent outbreaks during 1987–1996. *Harefuah.* **134**, 168–172, 248, 247.

Zhang-Wong, J. & Seeman, M. (2002). Antipsychotic drugs, menstrual regularity and osteoporosis risk. *Archives of Women's Mental Health.* **5**, 93–98.

Index